Athletic Strength
for Women

David Oliver
Dana Healy

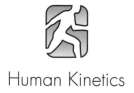

Human Kinetics

Library of Congress Cataloging-in-Publication Data

Oliver, David, 1964-
  Athletic strength for women / David Oliver, Dana Healy.
    p. cm.
  Includes bibliographical references and index.
  ISBN 0-7360-4632-1 (soft cover)
  1. Women athletes--Training of. 2. Sports for women--Physiological aspects. 3. Weight
training for women. I. Healy, Dana, 1972- II. Title.
  GV709.O55 2004
  613.7'1'082--dc22

                                                      2004010059

ISBN: 0-7360-4632-1

The Web addresses cited in this text were current as of January 3, 2005, unless otherwise noted.

Acquisitions Editor: Ed McNeely; **Developmental Editor:** Julie Rhoda; **Assistant Editor:** Carla Zych; **Copyeditor:** Annette Pierce; **Proofreader:** Kathy Bennett; **Indexer:** Nan N. Badgett; **Graphic Designer:** Nancy Rasmus; **Graphic Artist:** Tara Welsch; **Photo Manager:** Dan Wendt; **Cover Designer:** Keith Blomberg; **Photographer (cover):** © Tony Duffy; **Photographer (interior):** Tom Roberts, with the following exceptions: pp v (hurdler, swimmer), 1, 13, 17, 44, 58, 78 ©Sport the Library; pp v (field hockey player), 37, 97, 101, 143, 160 ©Empics; p 42 ©Human Kinetics; pp v (softball player), 139 ©Icon SMI; **Art Manager and Illustrator:** Kareema McLendon; **Printer:** United Graphics

We thank Oliver Sports in Orlando, Florida, for providing the location for the photo shoot for this book.

Human Kinetics books are available at special discounts for bulk purchase. Special editions or book excerpts can also be created to specification. For details, contact the Special Sales Manager at Human Kinetics.

Printed in the United States of America   10 9 8 7 6 5 4 3 2 1

Human Kinetics
Web site: www.HumanKinetics.com

United States: Human Kinetics
P.O. Box 5076
Champaign, IL 61825-5076
800-747-4457
e-mail: humank@hkusa.com

Canada: Human Kinetics
475 Devonshire Road Unit 100
Windsor, ON N8Y 2L5
800-465-7301 (in Canada only)
e-mail: orders@hkcanada.com

Europe: Human Kinetics
107 Bradford Road
Stanningley
Leeds LS28 6AT, United Kingdom
+44 (0) 113 255 5665
e-mail: hk@hkeurope.com

Australia: Human Kinetics
57A Price Avenue
Lower Mitcham, South Australia 5062
08 8277 1555
e-mail: liaw@hkaustralia.com

New Zealand: Human Kinetics
Division of Sports Distributors NZ Ltd.
P.O. Box 300 226 Albany
North Shore City
Auckland
0064 9 448 1207
e-mail: blairc@hknewz.com

Athletic Strength
for Women

Contents

Part IV   **Training for Performance**

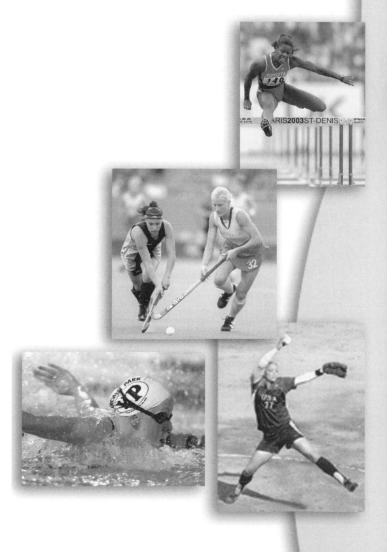

Acknowledgments

Thanks to my family—Shelly, Zachary, Ryan, Mom, and Dad.

Thanks to Lori, Seun, Nicole, Stacy, Brittany, Mo, and Christina for giving your time to make this possible.

And thanks to all my athletes and coaches for your inspiration through the years.

David Oliver

I would like to thank women in sport all over the world who have inspired this book. From youth sports to Olympic level competition, girls and women in sport have changed the way sport is perceived, accepted, and encouraged.

I also thank my colleagues at the Coaching and Sport Science Division, and the coaches and athletes at the United States Olympic Committee for the knowledge and experiences they have shared.

Dana Healy

Introduction

The opportunities for female athletes to compete at a high level have increased exponentially in recent years. We have seen a rapid increase in the number of athletes who participate in sport and in the number of sports available to young female athletes. And the opportunity to earn college scholarships has increased the level of play. Expanding the athlete pool has increased the physical demands—speed, agility, power, and skill—necessary to compete in each sport.

Although these significant changes in women's sport are happening, the training and conditioning programs needed to compete at these levels have not changed at the same pace. As the number of women participating in sport has increased, so too has the number of injuries sustained. During this same period, the injury rate for male athletes has not changed significantly. One reason is that many female athletes have increased the physical demands on their bodies without appropriately training their bodies' capacities to handle these demands. High school athletes are at greatest risk because often they lack basic strength training and speed training.

In particular, as female participation in sports has increased, we have seen epidemic levels of serious knee injuries such as ACL tears. Current research shows that including specific strength and power exercises may reduce the risk of injury. In this book we present performance-based and preventive programs that give athletes a significant performance advantage in their arena, while also helping to reduce the risk for serious injuries.

This book aims to provide the latest training methods and programs specific to the female athlete. Hundreds of books on strength, speed, flexibility, and power training cater to male athletes, but only a handful focus on the specific needs of women. We have spent much of our careers working with and catering to the specific needs of female athletes. We have worked with youth, high school, collegiate, professional, and Olympic-level athletes in a variety of sports—including field hockey, diving, soccer, gymnastics, lacrosse, and golf—and have gained the highest level of understanding of the real needs of these athletes. This book provides programs at different levels for conditioning and training female athletes for strength and power—from developing a simple base to working on explosiveness—while at the same time reducing the potential for injury. Along with our expertise we provide unique insights into training from some world-class athletes and coaches.

The book is divided into four parts. Part I, Setting the Stage, outlines the specific needs of female athletes through different developmental stages. Chapter 1 covers basic periodization principles that are the foundation of any year-round training program. Chapter 2, Assessing Your Potential, enables you to evaluate your current level of ability and helps you set goals based on a performance chart designed especially for female athletes. Coaches often ask us, "How do I gauge my athletes' sport-specific speed?" or "How do I measure my athletes' explosiveness?" Chapter 2 provides the tools needed to answer these questions.

Part II, Getting Stronger, identifies anatomical differences that predispose female athletes to risk of injury in the upper and lower body and in the core. The three chapters in this part focus on ways to prevent injuries with solid, basic strength-building exercises for the shoulder, hip, knee, ankle, and trunk regions. We often hear from coaches how their team's season was hampered by athlete injuries and the ensuing cutbacks in training. However, once their athletes start following a basic strength conditioning program—like the one outlined in these chapters—coaches begin to see how strength keeps athletes injury free. Whether you are a high school or elite athlete, decreasing your risk of injury allows you to continue training and therefore enhances your performance.

Part III, Gaining Power, may include the most significant chapters in this book. Once an athlete has laid the strengthening groundwork, she can use the information from these chapters to build the two skills necessary to perform at her peak—speed and power. (Strength and speed combined yield power.) Part III begins with a close look at stride technique in chapter 6, Strong Speed for Starting, Stopping, and Cutting. Chapter 7, Explosiveness for Jumping, Running, Throwing, and Striking, focuses on the proper lifting technique and progression for the Olympic lifts, plyometric exercises, and jumping mechanics. Chapter 7 also includes specific programs to enhance explosiveness that address the special needs of female athletes.

Part IV, Training for Performance, focuses on specific programs to improve performance using the exercises discussed throughout the book. Chapter 8 discusses a unique and effective way to warm up for each workout: The power warm-up goes beyond simply stretching and provides guidelines for increasing muscle temperature and nervous system efficiency while also working on technical performance. In chapter 9, you have access to a full season of workouts for your particular sport—each program is designed to improve strength and power for a specific sport. We provide ready-made exercise programs for basketball, diving, field hockey, golf, gymnastics, lacrosse, soccer, softball, sprinting, swimming, throwing, triathlon, and volleyball for preseason, in-season, and off-season training schedules.

This book is designed to give you a better understanding of training so that you can develop a cutting-edge strength and power program specifically for your needs. We provide accurate information about anatomy, physiology, and kinesiology, but keep it simple at the same time. Our goal is to give you the tools to design a proper training program that will increase your level of play while preventing injuries.

Exercise and Drill Finder

Exercise or drill	Page #	Test	Warm-up	Basket-ball	Diving	Field hockey	Golf	Gym-nastics	Lacrosse	Soccer	Softball	Swim-ming	Track sprints	Track throws	Triath-lon	Volley-ball
20-yard shuttle	29	X		X		X			X	X	X					X
20-yard sprint	28	X		X		X		X	X	X	X		X	X		X
40-yard sprint	29	X				X			X				X			
45-degree shoulder flexion	45			X	X	X	X	X	X	X	X	X		X	X	
300-yard shuttle	32	X		X		X		X	X	X	X		X	X	X	X
Abdominal curl	86			X	X	X	X	X	X	X	X	X	X	X	X	X
Ankle touch	85		X	X		X		X	X	X	X		X	X	X	X
Back raise	53			X	X	X	X	X	X	X	X	X	X	X	X	X
Back squat	65			X	X	X		X	X	X	X	X	X	X		X
Backward stride	162		X	X		X		X	X	X	X		X	X	X	X
Barrier strides	112			X		X		X	X	X	X		X		X	X
Bench obliques	86			X	X	X	X	X	X	X	X	X	X	X	X	X
Bench press	55			X	X	X	X	X	X	X	X	X	X	X	X	X
Body-weight shoulder stabiliza-tion routine	49			X	X	X	X	X	X	X	X	X		X		X
Bounding	113			X	X	X		X	X	X	X	X	X			X
Box jump for height	138			X	X			X				X				X
Box run shuffle	134			X		X		X	X	X	X		X			X
Box walk	54				X		X				X				X	
Bridge push-up	97				X		X	X				X				
Broad-jump test	28	X				X						X		X		

Exercise or drill	Page #	Test	Warm-up	Basketball	Diving	Field hockey	Golf	Gymnastics	Lacrosse	Soccer	Softball	Swimming	Track sprints	Track throws	Triathlon	Volleyball
Bungee sprints	115			X		X		X	X	X			X	X		
Bungee swing	57						X					X				
Calf stretch	156		X	X	X	X	X	X	X	X	X	X	X	X	X	X
Carioca	165		X	X		X		X	X	X	X		X	X		X
Chest pass on BOSU	104			X		X		X	X	X				X		X
Cutting drill	118		X	X		X			X	X	X					X
Cycle hops	142			X	X			X					X			X
Diagonal raise	50			X	X	X	X	X	X	X	X	X		X	X	X
Diagonal skating	117			X	X	X		X	X	X			X		X	X
Downhill running	116			X		X		X	X	X	X		X			
Dumbbell rotator cuff routine	44			X	X	X	X	X	X	X	X	X	X	X	X	X
Elbow bridge	99			X	X	X	X	X	X	X	X	X	X	X	X	X
Extended crunch	100			X	X	X	X	X	X	X	X	X	X	X	X	X
Extended crunch with pass	104			X	X	X		X	X	X					X	
External rotation	49			X	X	X	X	X	X	X	X	X		X	X	X
Fast-feet: backpedal	163		X	X		X			X	X	X					X
Fast-feet: forward	162		X	X		X		X	X	X	X		X			X
Fast-feet: forward, backward, forward	163		X	X		X			X	X	X					X
Fast-feet: sideways	163		X	X		X			X	X	X					X

Exercise or drill	Page #	Test	Warm-up	Sports used for (see program tables in chapter 9)												
				Basketball	Diving	Field hockey	Golf	Gymnastics	Lacrosse	Soccer	Softball	Swimming	Track sprints	Track throws	Triathlon	Volleyball
Forearm push-up	52											X				
Forearm side raise	53			X	X	X	X	X	X	X	X	X	X	X	X	X
Forward box step-up	73			X	X	X		X	X	X	X	X	X	X		X
Forward lunge stretch	154		X	X		X		X	X	X	X	X	X	X	X	X
Forward–backward leg swing	159		X	X		X		X	X	X	X	X	X	X	X	X
Front raise	46			X	X	X	X	X	X	X	X	X		X	X	X
Front squat	66			X							X	X	X	X		X
Front-to-back barrier hops	133			X	X	X		X	X	X	X		X			X
Full-ROM arm circles	161		X	X	X		X	X	X		X	X		X	X	X
Glute–ham: bent knee	92			X	X	X		X	X	X	X	X	X	X	X	X
Glute–ham: straight leg	71			X	X	X	X	X	X	X	X	X	X	X	X	X
Groin stretch	155		X	X	X	X	X	X	X	X	X	X	X	X	X	X
Hamstring stretch: straddle position	153		X	X	X	X	X	X	X	X	X	X	X	X	X	X
Handstand push-up	56				X			X								
Hang clean	127			X	X	X		X	X	X	X	X	X	X		X
Hanging knee raise	89			X	X	X	X	X	X	X	X	X	X	X	X	X

Exercise or drill	Page #	Test	Warm-up	Basketball	Diving	Field hockey	Golf	Gymnastics	Lacrosse	Soccer	Softball	Swimming	Track sprints	Track throws	Triathlon	Volleyball
								Sports used for (see program tables in chapter 9)								
Heel kick	164		X	X		X		X	X	X	X		X	X	X	X
High-knee skip	164		X	X		X		X	X	X	X		X	X	X	X
High pull	126			X	X	X			X	X	X		X	X	X	X
High pull from the floor	128								X		X			X		
Hip hike	99			X	X	X	X	X	X	X	X	X	X	X	X	X
Hyper-extension	102			X	X	X	X	X	X	X	X	X	X	X	X	X
I-drill	119	X		X		X			X	X						X
Iliotibial band stretch	154		X	X	X	X	X	X	X	X	X	X	X	X	X	X
Internal rotation	51			X	X	X	X	X	X	X	X	X		X	X	X
Jump rope drills	124			X				X			X		X	X		X
Knee–ankle swivel	160		X	X	X	X	X	X	X	X	X	X	X	X	X	X
Lat pull-down	56			X	X	X	X	X	X	X	X	X	X	X	X	X
Lateral box shuffle	140			X	X	X		X	X	X	X		X		X	X
Lateral raise	47			X	X	X	X	X	X	X	X	X		X	X	X
Latissimus dorsi stretch	157		X	X	X		X				X	X		X	X	X
Leg curl	103			X		X				X	X		X		X	X
Leg press with adduction	69						X									
Leger beep test	31	X		X		X			X	X						X
Medicine ball: chest pass	93			X	X	X	X	X	X	X	X		X		X	X

Exercise or drill	Page #	Test	Warm-up	Basket-ball	Diving	Field hockey	Golf	Gym-nastics	Lacrosse	Soccer	Softball	Swim-ming	Track sprints	Track throws	Triath-lon	Volley-ball
				Sports used for (see program tables in chapter 9)												
Medicine ball: over-head throw	95			X	X	X	X	X	X	X	X	X	X	X	X	X
Medicine ball: twist pass	94			X	X	X	X	X	X	X	X		X	X	X	X
Mile run	33	X		X		X			X	X		X			X	
No-step vertical leap	25	X		X	X	X		X	X	X	X	X	X	X		X
One-step vertical leap	26	X		X		X		X	X							X
Overhead side raise	48			X	X	X	X	X	X	X	X	X		X		X
Partner chest stretch	157		X	X							X	X		X		X
Physioball swimmer	58			X	X	X	X	X	X	X	X	X	X	X	X	X
Pike	98				X			X								
Pillars	96			X	X	X	X	X	X	X	X	X	X	X	X	X
Power clean	129										X			X		X
Power push-up	56				X			X							X	
Power shrug	125										X		X	X		X
Power skip	111			X	X			X						X		X
Prayer and seal stretches	158		X	X	X		X	X	X		X	X		X	X	X
Pull-up test	33	X		X		X		X	X			X		X	X	X
Push press	130			X	X	X		X		X	X	X	X	X		X
Push-up test	34	X		X		X		X	X	X	X	X		X	X	X
Quadri-ceps stretch	155		X	X	X	X	X	X	X	X	X	X	X	X	X	X

Exercise or drill	Page #	Test	Warm-up	Basketball	Diving	Field hockey	Golf	Gymnastics	Lacrosse	Soccer	Softball	Swimming	Track sprints	Track throws	Triathlon	Volleyball
				Sports used for (see program tables in chapter 9)												
Quick-response jump	135			X				X	X	X				X	X		X
Reverse crunch	90			X	X	X	X	X	X	X	X	X	X	X	X	X
Reverse hyperextension	101			X	X	X	X	X	X	X	X	X	X	X	X	X
Rice: three way	58			X		X	X	X	X		X					
Romanian deadlift	67			X	X	X		X	X	X	X	X	X	X		X
Seated row	57						X				X	X	X	X	X	X
Shoulder press	55			X							X	X	X	X		X
Shuffle squat	77														X	
Shuttle drill	119			X		X			X	X	X					X
Side box step-up	74			X	X	X		X	X	X	X					X
Side leg swing	159		X	X		X		X	X	X	X		X	X	X	X
Side lunge	75				X	X		X	X	X	X					
Side lunge stretch	153		X	X	X	X	X	X	X	X	X	X	X	X	X	X
Side-to-side barrier hops	133			X	X	X		X	X	X	X			X	X	X
Single-leg bounding	141			X	X	X		X	X	X	X			X	X	X
Single-leg hamstring curl	70											X				
Single-leg knee extension	70												X	X		X
Single-leg overhead throw	104			X			X	X	X	X				X		X

Part I

Setting the Stage

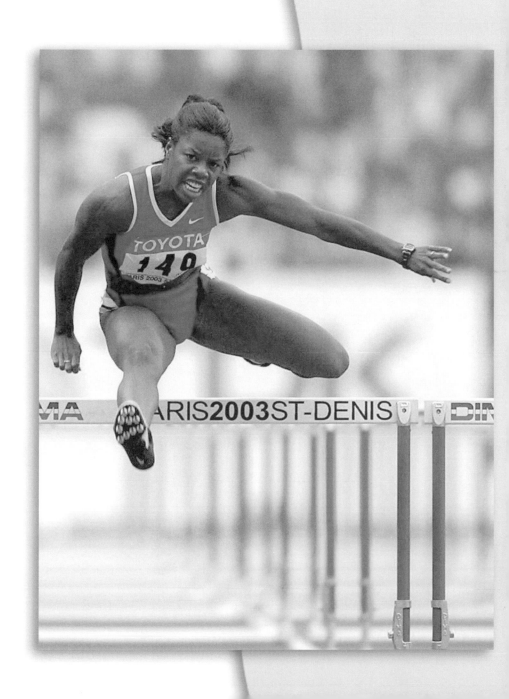

Laying the Foundation

Some say that athletes are born, not made. Although it may be true that not everyone can become an Olympic gymnast or volleyball player, anyone can become a good athlete. In becoming this type of athlete, it is necessary to take the proper steps to develop the body. The first step is choosing a sport. Most often, the sport finds the athlete rather than the other way around. You cannot change your body type or height. But you can determine which sports fit you and you can develop characteristics and skills over time that will enable you to become a better athlete.

Female athletes have made great strides, especially in the past decade, in athletic performance. Women are breaking records and smashing barriers. Female swimmers today are swimming faster than men were 10 years ago. Female sprinters continue to break speed records. Jumpers are clearing distances that were earlier thought unattainable by women. Female pitchers are striking out professional male baseball players, and tennis players are acing their male opponents. A female wrestler no longer has to wait in line to practice with the boys; wrestling was recently accepted as an Olympic sport for women.

How did this happen so quickly, in the past 10 to 15 years especially? Several factors explain and continue to contribute to these great improvements in athletic performance. Girls are being introduced to sport at an earlier age and therefore developing athletic characteristics at a younger age. Sport coaches are more knowledgeable about skills, technique, and physical preparation than ever before. Exercise science has come a long way and proved that women can train the same way men do. Not 50 years ago doctors suggested that female basketball athletes not run around the court, but just pass the ball, to keep from damaging their "female parts"!

Women now have the opportunity to work with strength and conditioning coaches to supplement their sport training. Strength and conditioning specialists use methods such as periodization to design long-term training plans that include resistance training, plyometrics, and metabolic conditioning as well as exercises to improve agility and flexibility, all in coordination with training for the specific sport. Elite athletes may spend up to six days a week for most of the year with a strength and conditioning coach, only taking time off immediately before competition or during breaks in training. The U.S. women's volleyball team follows its strength and conditioning plan up to three days prior to competition and begins again immediately after competition. The team takes time away from the court, but the athletes are expected to continue their resistance training and conditioning. This regimen helps prevent detraining and potential for injury.

Periodization is the scientific manipulation of training variables over periods within the training year to improve an athlete's overall fitness and performance in a specific sport. The result is the physical and physiological peak an athlete requires for competition. A periodized plan should be individualized for the athlete or team. That is where this book comes in—helping athletes and coaches plan a periodized training program to suit a particular athlete's or team's needs.

When training variables such as volume or amount, intensity, or focus are purposefully altered over periods, the athlete reduces her chance of overtraining. For example, if an athlete focuses only on strength work but not power training, she may overtrain certain muscle groups without reaping the benefits of power for her sport. When several training variables are systematically alternated throughout a period of training (as in periodization), a specific adaptation occurs without overstressing.

Training periods must progress step by step. Each period's training focus is achieved by altering several variables including volume, intensity, rest and recovery, and mode of training. But each phase also prepares the body for the next phase. For example, a sprinter might first develop her strength-endurance, then zero in on her strength, then add speed to achieve speed-strength or power, and finally fine-tune her speed. Each training phase builds on the previous training phase. This is called phase potentiation.

Although they are not covered in this book, programs that allow recovery and adaptation are another approach to periodization. This training principle is different from phase potentiation. Rather than training through a series of phases that build on each other, the athlete is overworked then allowed to recover within a training period. A typical example is a four-week training block. For three weeks the intensity increases, and the loading is expected to produce a negative effect on performance. On the fourth week, the load amount drops significantly, and the expected result is adaptation to the training stimulus and improved performance.

Let's take a look at some of the variables that form the basis for any periodized training program.

Volume is the number of sets and repetitions in a given training session. Repetitions are the number of times an exercise is performed within a set. Usually rest occurs only after the designated number of repetitions have been completed, not between each repetition. A set refers to the number of times each bundle of repetitions are completed. A designated rest time is allowed between each set of exercises. It can be manipulated in many different ways to achieve specific results. For example, an athlete may perform single sets (one set of 10 reps, or 1×10), multiple sets (3×10), pyramid sets ($1 \times 6, 1 \times 8, 1 \times 10, 1 \times 8, 1 \times 6$), super sets (where different exercises are done back-to-back without rest), and other combinations. Research suggests that multiple sets (three to six) produce the best overall results—significant increases in strength in both novice and elite athletes. And multiple sets allow for more variation, progression, and manipulation of volume to achieve the desired results. Typically, higher repetitions are used in the general preparation phase, and the volume decreases progressively as the athlete moves into the sport-specific and competition phases.

Intensity is the amount of work completed during a specific amount of time. Intensity can refer to both strength training and metabolic conditioning. In strength training, intensity is usually indicated by a percentage of the measured or predicted repetition maximum (RM). A percentage of maximal heart rate (HRmax) is most often used to determine intensity during conditioning sessions.

Rest and recovery allow the body to adapt to the stresses of training. Using appropriate rest and recovery methods and periods is just as important as the volume and intensity of the training program. Recovery is the rest period an athlete takes between sets, training sessions, or training periods. A shorter rest period between sets of exercises promotes muscular endurance, higher heart rates, and some cardiovascular enhancement. Shorter rest periods are included in the general preparation phase to promote muscular endurance and basic fitness. These periods may last 15 seconds to one minute. Longer rest periods, two to three minutes, allow for greater recovery, which promotes increased reproduction of adenosine triphosphate (ATP), the fuel for muscle actions. When developing speed and power, use longer rest periods to maximize neural adaptation. If an athlete doesn't allow adequate recovery between sets and training sessions, the neuromuscular system may not adapt as it should. Volume, intensity, and rest must be combined properly to avoid negative training effects. Athletes are stressed and pushed beyond normal levels of activity during training sessions. How an athlete recovers and adapts depends not only on the appropriate loading and rest, but also on outside stressors such as school, social activity, travel, work, nutrition, sleep patterns, and the environment. The recovery period, in addition to proper nutrition and sleep, allows the body to regenerate and build.

Mode of training refers to the exercises and equipment chosen for the training program. The exercises dictate what the training response will be. For example, while a leg extension completed on a resistance machine and a box step-up both focus on strengthening the quadriceps, each mode delivers slightly different results. Traditional resistance machines (e.g., leg curl, chest press, row, and leg press) strengthen one or more muscle groups in one plane of movement Thus, these machines are best for training isolated muscle groups and achieving balance between muscle groups. Free weights are considered optimal over resistance machines for training athletes for sports because the movement of the resistance can occur in several planes and at various speeds, just like during sports movements. For example, the athlete must also use the legs and trunk to stabilize the body while performing a standing shoulder press. This simulates sport movements more than a seated shoulder press on a machine, which works only the shoulder muscles. The shoulders need to maintain stability while a dynamic contraction is completed.

Olympic weightlifting (see chapter 7) is considered one of the most sport-specific resistance training forms. Exercises such as the power clean require strength, speed, coordination, flexibility, and balance. Plyometrics (see chapter 7) are a form of speed training especially good for developing explosiveness. Usually body weight provides the only resistance. Ballistic movements like jumping and throwing develop quick reaction and response (see chapter 7). An athlete or coach must carefully consider the desired outcome before determining the mode of exercise that best achieves the goals of the program. This book and the program tables in chapter 9 will help you determine which particular exercises are appropriate for your sport.

The three general phases in a periodized cycle are: general preparation, specific preparation, and competition. A fourth phase, called the transitional phase, is a short period that allows recovery after the competition phase. When planned correctly, these phases coincide with an athlete's sport-specific training and competitive seasons and form the basis for the overall training plan. The succession of these phases completes a single macrocycle. The **macrocycle** usually lasts 12 months, but can be longer or shorter to account for the duration of an athlete's season. A **mesocycle** is a shorter period within the macrocycle, often corresponding to one of the phases. A mesocycle or phase usually lasts 12 or more weeks. Figure 1.1 shows generally how a macrocycle and its mesocycles might be structured around a competitive season. Notice how the variables of intensity and volume vary throughout the training year and within each training phase. Table 1.1 also shows how volume, intensity, and frequency of workouts might vary throughout each mesocycle of training.

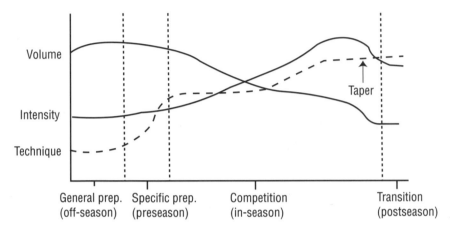

General prep.   Specific prep.   Competition   Transition
(off-season)   (preseason)   (in-season)   (postseason)

Figure 1.1 A macrocycle for sport is made up of smaller units called mesocycles.

Table 1.1 General Periodization for Strength and Power Training

	Mesocycles			
Variable	General preparation (strength-endurance)	Specific preparation (basic strength)	Competition (strength and power)	Transition
Intensity	Low to moderate	High	High to very high	Low
Repetition	High (8-20)	Moderate to high (4-6)	Low (2-3)	Very low (1-3)
Sets	3-5	3-5	4-5	1-3
Days/week	3-6	3-5	2-4	3

Within each mesocycle are weekly cycles with very specific goals. These are called microcycles. A **microcycle** allows the coach to predetermine which training variables best match the sport training and meet the specific goals of the strength and conditioning plan. As with the microcycles, the workouts within a microcycle are structured with variable intensities and volumes to allow the athlete to effectively recover and adapt to the training (see figure 1.2). For example a heavy lifting day should not precede a practice that will focus on skill and technique because the athlete will not be sufficiently recovered from the lifting to produce high quality efforts when practicing the skill and technique drills.

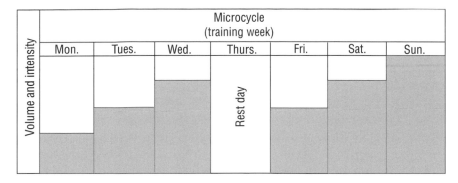

Figure 1.2 A mesocycle is made up of microcycles. Each microcycle has a specific goal.

GENERAL PREPARATION PHASE: OFF-SEASON

All successful strength and conditioning programs set intermediate training goals throughout the training year. Whether the goal is to develop power, speed, or strength, every program should begin with a solid general preparation or base-producing phase. This phase is as essential to the novice as it is to the elite athlete. General base training prepares the body for sport-specific strength and power training. Training programs should slowly and progressively strengthen tendons and ligaments, promote bone density, and increase blood flow to working muscles, which may induce hypertrophy (an increase of muscle size). These effects play an integral role in preparing the body for the high-intensity demands that will come with in-season training and competition.

The most appropriate time for base training or general preparation is during the off-season. The general preparation phase may be the most important period because it provides the foundational strength for the later development of power. General strength and conditioning, through the creation of a strong core, stable shoulders, and stable hips, knees, and ankles are the focus of this phase. Volume and intensity are inversely related during this period. The volume of exercises, or number of sets and repetitions, is usually moderate to high to encourage muscular endurance, while the intensity is low to allow adequate recovery and to prevent overtraining.

We encourage athletes to complete several weeks of base training before undergoing physical testing. Athletes who test their fitness without any strength training may be susceptible to injury. However, testing an athlete after the first phase of training is a safe way to establish a base reading for the athlete's physical condition (see chapter 2).

The duration and intensity of the base phase depends largely on the amount of time before the preseason begins. We recommend that athletes spend at least 12 weeks for this training phase. For example, if a basketball player's preseason practices start in October, she might start her base training in August or earlier in the summer. Most athletes have longer off-season periods than in-season. This off-season allows ample time to build base strength.

Of course, fitting in an adequate base-training phase can be most challenging for the multisport high school athlete and the amateur elite athlete. The summer months may be the only time a high school athlete can establish a base of training that will take her through the entire school year. She should use these few months to her advantage to prepare her general conditioning.

To prepare the body physically for a specific sport, it is important to include multi-joint and multidirectional exercises throughout the base-training phase. This phase is often misunderstood and associated with slow, single-joint movements. Although these exercises can and should be included in the base program, coaches and athletes must remember that most sport movements are multidirectional and explosive.

The exercises you choose should depend on your level and experience. Early in the general preparation phase, focus on core training, joint stability, and proprioception training. Proprioception refers to an athlete's awareness of her body in space and sense of balance. Core training includes work on the abdominals and low back as its cornerstone. Squats and weightlifting movements such as pulls, power cleans, and push presses (see chapter 7) are also essential to the base program. These multijoint movements strengthen and increase flexibility of the shoulder, low back, hip, knee, and ankle joints. Complex movements encourage balance and proprioception. Other drills include single- or double-leg movements on an unstable surface such as an air-filled pillow or foam roller. The goal is to place stress on the body both physically and physiologically.

The shoulder is one of the areas most prone to injury and overuse. A combination of low- and high-speed movements that isolate the small muscles surrounding the joint can protect and help prevent injuries to the supporting girdle of the shoulder. Chapter 3 provides specific exercises to help develop stability in the shoulder joint.

The knee joint is extremely prone to catastrophic injuries such as ligament and meniscus tears and patella tracking problems in the female athlete. Muscle imbalance is the common culprit because the quadriceps muscles tend to overdevelop compared to the hamstring group. Developing quadriceps and hamstring muscle balance while focusing on correct linear movement and knee stability during flexion and extension can provide female athletes with protection against knee injuries. During the general preparation phase, an athlete should master forward and backward movement first, followed by lateral movements.

The ankle joint is one of the most efficient joints in the body. A simple standing ankle extension easily lifts the entire body weight. Yet as strong and stable as it appears, the joint is a complex combination of tendons, ligaments, and bones so close to the playing surface that it is an easy target for injuries. Soccer requires quick changes of direction that place great amounts of stress on the ankle. Team sports like volleyball and basketball often result in collisions that lead to tripping or landing improperly. To prepare the joint for these types of movements and occurrences, the athlete should train the supporting structures of the ankle through multidirectional concentric (flexing) and eccentric (extending) contractions. Standing barefoot on equipment that provides unstable surfaces encourages balance, proprioception, and strength. Chapter 4 covers exercises that strengthen the hip, knee, and ankle joints.

You can also incorporate low-level plyometrics, agility drills, and sprint mechanics (see part III) into this general preparation program to prepare you for moderate to intense training. Jump rope, double-leg jumps, and form running are good exercises for beginners to start with. Each of these exercises is detailed in this book, and samples of full programs for various sports are provided in chapter 9.

Conditioning during the general preparation phase should correspond to the strength training program. You'll design the conditioning program to prepare your body for the sport-specific training you will do throughout the rest of the training year. Aerobic conditioning and interval training provide a conditioning base to build on. During the general preparation phase, you'll keep aerobic intensity moderate, 60 to 75 percent of one RM for strength training and 50 to 70 percent of your HRmax for aerobic training.

SPECIFIC PREPARATION PHASE: PRESEASON

The specific preparation phase is often called preseason training. During this phase, strength training and power training become more specific to the sport. This phase may be included as a separate mesocycle or part of a mesocycle and may last 12 or more weeks. This phase focuses on sport-specific drills and conditioning. Foundational exercises, which were the focus of the general preparation phase, are still part of the program but take on a secondary role. An athlete attends to individual weaknesses and needs during this phase. We recommend that athletes perform an assessment at the beginning and at the end of this phase (see chapter 2 for full assessment details). This allows the coach to determine the effectiveness of the current training program and assists in providing new goals for the athlete.

The relationship between volume and intensity changes as the athlete shifts from the general preparation phase to this phase (refer to figure 1.1). Intensity now increases to promote speed and power. This can be done in one of three ways. The most general and widely used method is to decrease the training volume and increase the training intensity. The program may keep the volume steady and vary the intensity, or maintain the intensity and vary the volume. During the specific preparation phase, intensity may increase to 75 to 90 percent for strength training. Depending on the metabolic characteristics of the sport, the intensity for aerobic conditioning may increase from what it was during the general preparation phase or fluctuate to induce the appropriate adaptations. An endurance athlete's program may include interval training, while a program for an athlete in a sport that requires short bursts may include sprint work at intensities of up to 100 percent.

One pitfall to avoid during the preseason is overtraining. Maintaining a high level of intensity or volume over a long period may not allow adequate recovery. During this phase, the intensity and volume increase throughout. Recovery periods become very important. As the training load increases, the need for proper recovery and rest also increases. The specific program tables for various sports in chapter 9 provide proper guidelines to ensure enough recovery to help prevent overtraining.

During the specific preparation phase, the number of exercises decreases and the exercises become more specific. The Olympic lifts are major players for power and speed sports during this phase. Exercises such as the hang clean, high pull, and power shrug are best. Throughout this phase you train the neuromuscular system to produce high levels of force through a combination of heavy strength exercises and speed drills. For endurance sports, the focus is on drills that improve economy and efficiency and exercises that prevent injury. Drills that improve economy and efficiency increase the rate of force (how much the neurological and muscular systems work together) and propulsion time, and decrease the potential for fatigue.

COMPETITION PHASE: IN-SEASON

As the competitive season begins, it is time to shift the emphasis away from training and toward sport performance. To the extent allowed by the length of the season, training sessions must be incorporated to maintain the power levels developed during the specific preparation phase. During the competition phase, a fine line separates overtaxing the neuromuscular system and not training enough to maintain the levels achieved during earlier phases. Detraining, or losing the effects of training, can occur within 72 hours if the athlete does not train regularly; therefore, it is important to

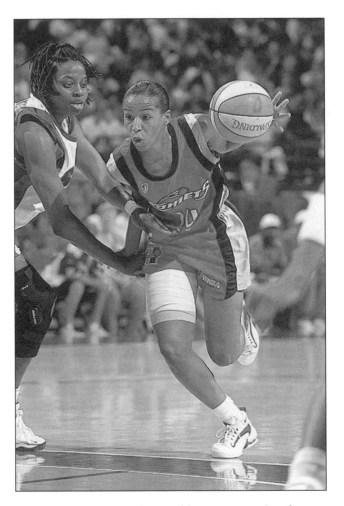

During the competition phase, athletes maintain their fitness and sport skills through low-volume, high-quality training.

continue training throughout the season. The most effective method is a combination of sport-specific drills. Volume is considerably lower than in prior phases. Intensity and rest remain high. Supplemental secondary exercises are added individually based on need.

During the general preparation phase, volume and intensity were inversely related. The same is true with in-season training; however, the emphasis is opposite. During in-season training, the volume is low while the intensity increases to its highest level to focus on power and speed. During the competition phase, intensity is adjusted to meet the needs of competition. The intensity may increase or stay the same as the volume of drills and exercises changes. The competition phase is not a training period, but a maintenance period. The time spent in the weight room decreases as more time is spent perfecting skills, plays, and technique for competition. The variables fluctuate during the competition phase to prevent overtraining and avoid staleness. Quality is most important during the competition phase. Each repetition should be of the highest quality. If the rest period does not allow for complete recovery, performance will likely deteriorate and result in the development of improper neural patterns; this is similar to learning a skill incorrectly. It will take a great amount of time to relearn the proper patterns. Again, chapter 9 details how to train appropriately during this phase for your specific sport.

TRANSITION PHASE: POSTSEASON

Every athlete needs time to unwind from the competitive season and to rest before the start of the next general preparation period. At this time the athlete can and should take time away from her sport, doing other things to stay active while taking a break. This phase should include active recovery. We do not suggest sitting on the couch for three months, but rather participating in activities that promote basic conditioning and fitness at a casual level. This phase should be fun, and the intensity is low.

AGE-APPROPRIATE PERIODIZED TRAINING

Consider each athlete individually when designing a training program. How an athlete adapts to training depends on her athletic experience and physical maturity, as well as her chronological age. One can expect a novice athlete to demonstrate greater improvements compared to an elite athlete. Physiological age plays a similar role. Two 15-year-old girls may adapt at different rates because of individual physiological and physical maturation rates as well as individual differences in their experience level in the sport. The trainability of an athlete and her intrinsic motivation are psychological factors that will speed or slow adaptation. A training program should reflect the athlete's personal characteristics.

Several professional organizations including the National Strength and Conditioning Association (NSCA), the American Academy of Pediatrics (AAP), and the American College of Sports Medicine (ASCM) have set guidelines for determining when a child is ready for strength training. These guidelines can help parents and coaches decide if a child should start formal training and what type of training would be best for her age, maturity, and activity level. These guidelines are conservative and are based on scientific research. Taking the right steps in training girls and young women over time may be the best preparation for a lifetime of sport and activity. Starting as young as three or four with general play for coordination and balance, and progressively challenging the developing child builds not only strong bones and muscles, but also the confidence to become a better athlete.

Preschool and Elementary School–Age Girls (Ages 3 to 8)

Developing strength and power starts far before making the varsity basketball team. It starts with a lifetime of play and physical activity. All young girls should be encouraged to be physically active at a young age. Play may be the best form of activity because it encourages a healthy lifestyle and the healthy habits that foster a strong body. Formal strength training is not recommended for girls this young.

Play can include organized and unorganized activities. Both help develop a foundation that a future athlete can build on and rely on. Even general play develops strength, coordination, and balance—the building blocks of power.

Organized activities offer girls the chance to learn new skills and challenge themselves in a supervised environment. Tumbling, gymnastics, swimming, martial arts, dance, soccer, and T-ball are just a few examples of common organized activities. Local clubs and organizations such as the Young Men's Christian Association (YMCA), Young Women's Christian Association (YWCA), Boys and Girls Clubs of America (BGCA), and the Girl Scouts of America (GSA) may also provide programs for young children. Participating in these programs is a great way to combine physical activity and other activities in a team environment.

Another advantage to organized activities is the presence of an adult leader, usually one who knows how children adapt to physical activity and stress and can provide proper instruction, guidance, and motivation in a safe environment. An instructor-to-athlete ratio of at least 1 to 10 is recommended to provide adequate supervision and instruction. Sometimes more instructors are necessary when young children are learning skills for the first time. The facility where these activities take place should be free of hazards, well lit, and ventilated. Adequate fluids should be available, and children should be encouraged to drink throughout the activity. The programs should focus on the girls having fun and enjoying the challenge of physical activity in a safe environment. How the child perceives physical activity will play an important role in her athletic future.

Unorganized activity is also important, and its only downfall is its frequent lack of supervision. Adult supervision and a safe environment are also important in unorganized activities. Children learn best by doing or mimicking an action; therefore, sport-related games or skills should be played with parents or siblings who can model proper technique as well as anticipate safety problems or detect when play is getting out of hand and becoming dangerous. When supervising children, adults should treat them with respect, and speak to them in language they can understand. Children should feel comfortable with the activity and look forward to doing it again.

Prepubescent Girls (Ages 8 to 12)

As girls mature in age and experience, the introduction to sports and organized activities is often the next step. A young athlete has many choices besides traditional strength training to enhance her fitness and potential for athletic ability. Although unorganized activities benefit athletes at this age, organized activities are often superior because they are supervised and provide a supportive environment.

A formal introduction to strength and conditioning is best between the ages of 7 and 12, keeping in mind that age is usually not the best indicator of readiness. Physical maturity is often a better indicator of when a child can begin this type of training and how much she can handle. As with teaching skills, a slow progressive approach is the best way to start strength training and conditioning. This age group demonstrates various levels of readiness. The training volume and intensity should be carefully monitored to keep from overloading the athlete. Each session should begin with a progressive warm-up and simple stretching to prepare the body for the training ahead.

Athletes in this age group who participate in organized activity may have the option of including strength training in their overall training plan. In addition to enhancing muscular strength and endurance, a properly designed and followed program can reduce the risk of injury. Strength sessions should always be supervised and should take place in a safe facility. An adult, preferably a certified strength training professional, is the best supervisor and can help set goals and develop a program that is safe and progressive and appropriate for the young athlete's needs. Note that training prepubescent athletes under proper supervision has been shown to increase strength. However, studies have not proven that the increased strength enhances their performance.

Strength exercises that focus on large muscle groups, for instance the large muscles of the legs—the hamstrings and quadriceps—are a great place to start. You should also include other large muscles, such as the back, abdominals, and chest. Basic exercises that can be performed using body weight only at first and using free weights such as dumbbells and barbells later are preferred, but exercises done on resistance machines are also a good way to develop strength. Free weights are preferred because they help develop other athletic qualities such as balance and coordination and using the entire body during exercises. Maximal lifting is not recommended for this age group. Exercises should be submaximal and train the muscles and ligaments to withstand this level of stress. This prepares the joints and muscles for more specific and heavier loading when it's appropriate.

Adhere to periodization principles when training pubescent and postpubescent athletes. Not only is physical maturity important at this age, but so is psychological maturity. Keep in mind that at the high school level, peer pressure exists even in

12

the weight room. Athletes of lesser physical maturity may feel pressed to train at an inappropriately high level, resulting in serious injury or even death. Supervision by a qualified and certified coach is absolutely necessary to maintain safety. Novice lifters should begin with a total-body workout consisting of one set of 10 to 15 repetitions for each major muscle group. It is best to begin with a light load that slightly stresses the body. Keep detailed records of each workout to help set new goals and design new programs. Examples of programs appropriate for novice lifters are provided later in the book.

Adolescent Girls (Ages 13 to 18)

After puberty, a young woman's body undergoes many changes, including changes in the way she adapts to physical training. As a girl reaches the age and maturity level to physically withstand higher-intensity strength training, she can begin more traditional methods of athletic preparation.

As a female athlete reaches adolescence, it may become important to choose a training facility that fits her needs. At this age the athlete has more choices in where and how she will train. Some high schools have strength training equipment available at little or no cost and may be the most economical. But the facility should meet the same standards required of a commercial gym. It should be safe and clean and should provide appropriate, well-maintained equipment as well as appropriate supervision. As with lifting for younger girls, free weights are preferred over resistance machines. Access to the facility should be convenient for the athlete and should allow adequate time to complete a workout. Fluids should be available for the athlete, or she should plan to bring them with her to maintain proper hydration.

A commercial gym is usually focused on making a profit and therefore is sometimes an expensive alternative. Athletes should remember that although basic equipment and facilities are required, fancy equipment and gimmicks are not. Choose a commercial gym that offers what you need, allows you to feel comfortable, and provides educated and competent supervision that is readily available when you could use a hand or have a question. The benefits of a commercial gym are the hours of operation, wide variety of equipment, and certified staff.

Some young athletes have the option of training at home, where their parents have set up a home gym. Although this is convenient, it is not the best choice for young female athletes. No one requires the equipment to be maintained regularly or checks to make sure ventilation is appropriate. Most important, supervision is often lacking. The home gym can become a dangerous place even when training with a partner or parent. Only the most experienced parent with extensive knowledge should supervise a young athlete in a home gym.

Postadolescent Girls and Adults (Ages 19 and Older)

Training for more mature athletes uses the same strength program periodization and planning. However, some training aspects will and should change. As a young female matures, she also becomes more serious about her sport and abilities as an athlete. High school, club, and collegiate sports have become very competitive as female athletes have become stronger, faster, and more powerful. As sports like women's wrestling are being accepted, not only by the general public but also as an Olympic event, opportunities in competitive sports have been blown wide open. While opportunities have increased, so too have the number of women participating. Along with the increased opportunity and increased participation has come further pressure to be stronger, faster, and more powerful in order to compete effectively.

Following a strict program to develop sport-specific athleticism takes time, dedication, and motivation. While training should still be fun, it is more serious at this level. Specific warm-ups, plyometrics, speed training, resistance training, and conditioning all play a role. Each component is pieced together to achieve the desired result.

Sample programs for specific sports are provided later in this book. These programs are guidelines and should be tailored to meet each athlete's specific needs. Three or four days of training per week are recommended, using sets of three or more for each exercise. Multijoint exercises such as squats and hang cleans should be a basic component of the program. These exercises and many others are described in detail in the chapters that follow.

At the postadolescent level of training, supervision is extremely important, just as it is at any level. However, at this level of competition and training, whom you choose to supervise the training becomes more important. Options include the sport coach, strength coach, personal trainer, athletic trainer, and training partner. Each person will offer a strength, and based on who is available, the athlete must decide who is most knowledgeable, will motivate her, and will maintain safety. For strength training purposes, it's best to work with a certified and experienced strength and conditioning coach. This person should know the sport, be certified in cardiopulmonary resuscitation (CPR), and know the athlete's needs and goals. Although the strength and conditioning coach is best suited to supervise strength sessions, it takes the whole support staff to determine what the athlete needs and how best to achieve it. Collaborative effort by the relevant parties provides the best support for the athlete. The flow of communication to and from the athlete should also flow to and from the team around the athlete.

The training plan should be based on comprehensive analysis from each party. The strength and conditioning coach should evaluate the athlete. The athlete can also evaluate herself. This evaluation should include strength training experience, general strengths and weaknesses, injury history, information specific to the sport, and any other important information. Chapter 2 provides several evaluation tests that can help the coach and athlete put together an appropriate training plan.

The final components of a sound training program are time management and rest. High school and collegiate athletes are usually very active and need to schedule time for rest and recovery. Training is no good without recovery, which includes rest and proper nutrition. A balanced athlete is the best athlete. Overloading athletes with training programs that are too demanding can produce negative results. The training program should include the right combination of ingredients added at the right time at the right rate. This book will help you create your own recipe for success.

Assessing Your Potential

Much of this chapter lays the groundwork for understanding where an athlete's fitness or conditioning has been, where it is now, and how much potential she has for improving her athletic performance. Athletes can perform general sport evaluation tests at the start of the season and throughout the season to determine what their strengths are as well as what aspects of their training they need to focus on.

It is true that physiological differences between men and women create a gap in performance potential and injury rates. However, the gap is narrowing in all aspects of sport. After working with the U.S. women's national soccer team from 1997 to 2000 and the U.S. women's national basketball team from 1999 to 2000, there is no doubt in our minds that young female athletes have the potential for great performances. Almost all of the athletes at this level produced test results that surpassed our expectations. Significant improvement comes more slowly to elite athletes than to less-experienced athletes, yet these teams showed marked improvement with each testing session. The quality that stands out in these women is their commitment to excellence. They never settled for second best or compromised in any way. They set a standard for all athletes—women and men alike.

Before starting any training regimen, you or your coach must understand where you are and where you want to go. Moreover, it is helpful to be able to measure your progress objectively throughout a season as well as from season to season. This is where periodic athletic testing comes in.

You'll complete an initial test at the start of your preseason training; that is, after you have completed basic conditioning during the off-season or general preparation phase (see chapter 1). Because of the physical nature of many of these tests, it is important to engage in a general preparation conditioning program, ideally for 12 weeks but minimally for 3 weeks, before undergoing this testing. General conditioning will gradually build your fitness and decrease the likelihood of injury during testing. Moreover, as you follow the programs outlined in chapter 9, you'll see that general conditioning also includes exercises that simulate some of the tests you will perform, which further prepares your body for the tests and prevents injuries. For example, before testing we recommend that you add 300-yard shuttle runs at 75 percent of your maximum speed (submaximal performance), broad jumps, or 20-yard shuttles. Adding these exercises to your training beforehand will familiarize you with the specific tests you will perform.

You'll likely want to repeat the testing at the end of the preseason phase to see how you or your team has progressed through preseason training. If your preseason phase is long enough, you may choose to test in the middle of it and use the testing data to evaluate how well your training is contributing to gains in skill level.

The testing format we present is similar to the one we used with the national basketball and soccer programs. It can be used for most sports at the high school, collegiate, and professional levels to measure athletic ability and to set goals for future development. Coaches and trainers can use these tests to evaluate athletes at all levels of sport and can select the tests that are most specific to certain sports. The resulting data can be used to help an athlete improve her athleticism and therefore her performance. In many cases the results may be used to evaluate an athlete's ability to play at the next level (collegiate or professional). The information we present in this chapter is a compilation of more than 12 years of data we have collected from athletes at all levels and abilities.

WHAT TO TEST

Before testing, you must determine the reason for performing a test or sequence of tests and the methods you will use. For example, when testing basketball players for speed, you don't need to test them on a 40-yard sprint because the court is not 40-yards long, so instead test them for 20 yards. A swimmer or diver would not perform a three-hop test, which tests quickness, balance upon landing, and explosiveness, but these athletes might instead perform a no-step vertical leap to measure pure power (similar to coming off the block in a swimming start or coming off the platform for a dive).

Understanding what you are measuring and why you are testing a certain skill for a particular sport is essential for knowing how to use the data. When we test individuals and teams, we typically try to create a profile for overall athleticism. A person with overall athleticism almost always possesses more than one of the following traits. Refer to the following definitions to help you better understand which skills or aspects of sport you want to measure.

Speed is defined as the rate of performance, shown by the ratio of work done to time spent. Simply put, speed is how fast you move from point A to B. You can measure the speed of something moving in a straight line or of something changing direction. Speed, like strength, can be developed in every athlete through technical and physical training.

Acceleration refers to the rate at which the velocity of a body increases per unit of time. A person with great acceleration gets to top-end speed very quickly. Usually those who accelerate at a rapid rate can also produce great speed. Coaches often confuse acceleration with speed, but as you can see, each is defined differently.

Strength (of the upper and lower body) refers to the athlete's ability to move a mass without considering the time it takes to move the mass. Coaches typically refer to several types of strength. Pure or absolute strength refers to the ability to move a maximal weight. Strength-endurance (also called muscular endurance) refers to the athlete's ability to move a mass repeatedly for a maximal amount of time.

Power refers to a combination of strength and speed. Many coaches define power as strength times speed. In order for an athlete to maximize her power, she must improve her strength. Power is defined as the rate at which energy is transferred into work. The tests measure power in several ways. We measure pure vertical power (no-step jump) and vertical power with momentum (one-step jump). We also administer a power test that incorporates balance and coordination. Coaches also often confuse strength with power.

Agility is the combination of several athletic traits including speed, power, strength, and coordination. Agility is maximized if the athlete possesses each of these traits. Most sports require athletes to move multidirectionally and require athletes to maximize their agility. The tests in this book measure both lateral and multidirectional agility.

Cardiovascular endurance is measured in what sport scientists refer to as $\dot{V}O_2$max. $\dot{V}O_2$max is the efficiency at which an athlete uses oxygen (O_2) to create energy for work. $\dot{V}$ refers to the volume of O_2 the body can take up. An athlete whose body takes up and uses more O_2 is able to perform at a higher level for a longer amount of time than someone with a lower $\dot{V}O_2$max. Endurance testing uses longer bouts of exercise than the other tests.

Lactate threshold is the point during exercise of increasing intensity at which lactate from the muscles begins to accumulate in the blood faster than it can be cleared. Tests that measure this point are typically the most difficult and most hated by athletes. Lactic acid (lactate) is produced in muscles during intense bouts of exercise where the heart rate is driven beyond its aerobic level. When this occurs the muscles produce lactate, and the body feels a "heavy burning" sensation. These tests are important for sports like basketball, soccer, field hockey, lacrosse, hockey, tennis, and others that involve repetitive bouts of intense work followed by short rest.

Flexibility determines a joint's range of motion, or how far the muscle allows a bone to move around a joint. Testing flexibility is difficult and not always as precise as we would like it to be, but nonetheless, it is important to look at an athlete's preprogram and postprogram flexibility. Improvements in range of motion can lead to improvements in performance and a decrease in injury rates.

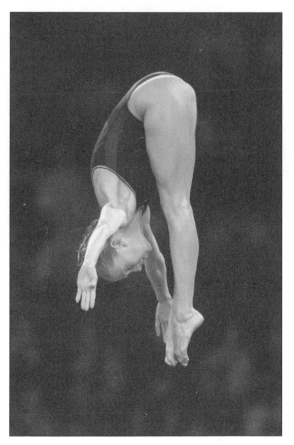

Sports such as diving demand great strength and flexibility while others rely more on power.

Use these definitions along with an understanding of the physiological demands of your sport to devise and perform testing that measures the traits that are most relevant. Table 2.1 provides an example of several sports and their recommended testing schedules. The table lists tests for different categories of athleticism (for example, power and speed) and indicates which tests are appropriate for each sport. Each category offers multiple test choices. An athlete or coach should not pick all of the tests in a category, but select one or two from each category that are appropriate.

At the bottom of table 2.1 you will notice a sport-specific testing category. Sport-specific tests are those that you already use for your sport and want to continue using. For example, sports like golf require very specific testing regarding the golf swing, however, such specific tests are outside the scope of this book.

HOW TO TEST

Once you have selected the tests you will perform, follow these basic testing guidelines to ensure accurate data collection.

- Perform a general warm-up and stretching routine before testing. A proper warm-up may include jogging or jumping rope for five minutes, a general full-body stretch (see chapter 8), and 5 to 10 minutes of speed or movement drills (see chapter 8).

Table 2.1 Sample Testing Profile for Various Sports

	Test	Basketball	Soccer	Volleyball	Softball	Lacrosse or field hockey
Power	No-step vertical leap	X	X	X	X	X
	One-step vertical leap	X	X	X		X
	Three-hop test	X	X	X	X	X
	Broad-jump test					
Speed and acceleration	20-yd sprint	X	X	X	X	X
	40-yd sprint		X			X
Agility	20-yd shuttle	X	X	X	X	X
	T-test	X	X	X	X	X
Endurance and lactate threshold	Leger beep test	X	X	X		X
	300-yd shuttle	X	X	X	X	X
	Mile run	X	X			X
Strength	Push-up test	X	X	X	X	X
	Pull-up test	X		X		X
	Sit-up test	X	X	X	X	X
Flexibility	Sit-and-reach test	X	X	X	X	X
Sport-specific	Depends on sport	X	X	X	X	X

- Perform flexibility testing next.
- Perform short, explosive tests next.
- Perform speed and agility testing.
- Perform endurance tests last.
- Perform strength testing on a separate day.

If you have selected more than five tests for your sport, perform the testing over two separate days to ensure safety and accurate test data. For example, if you are testing your high school basketball team and have chosen to test the one-step vertical leap, no-step vertical leap, 20-yard sprint, 20-yard shuttle, 300-yard shuttle, Leger beep test, push-up test, sit-and-reach test, sit-up test, and three-hop test you might divide your testing as follows:

Day 1	Day 2
Warm-up	Warm-up
Sit-and-reach test	20-yard shuttle
Vertical leap (no step or one step)	300-yard shuttle
Three-hop test	Sit-up test
20-yard sprint	Push-up test
Leger beep test	

Gymnastics	Triathlon	Golf	Diving	Track (field events)	Track (running events)	Swimming
X			X	X	X (sprinters)	X
X					X (sprinters)	
		X	X			X
X				X	X (for starts)	
					X (100 m)	
X	X			X	X (200, 400 m)	
	X				X (1500 to 3000 m)	X
X	X			X		X
X	X			X		X
X	X	X	X	X	X	X
X	X	X	X	X		
X	5K, 10K time trials	X		Jumps, throws, lifts as appropriate		

To ensure accuracy whenever you retest, perform the same exercises in the same sequence under the same conditions, if possible. For example, conduct the tests at the same time of day and in the same weather conditions.

EVALUATING YOUR TEST SCORES

Once you have completed the battery of tests, you can use the scores and the points system to evaluate your strengths and weaknesses. The scores are provided in the tables that accompany each test description (see page 25 for an example of a table that shows both raw scores and points). Please note, however, that this system is meant to provide a positive tool for assessment and motivation. Coaches should use these tests for team and individual improvement rather than for disqualification, especially at the high school level.

The values listed in the raw score column for each test are based on averages taken from athletes in all sports. We know, for example, that a basketball player's vertical leap will likely be higher than that of a softball player, and should be, but the numbers are all relative to the female athlete depending on her level of development (i.e., whether she is a high school athlete, college athlete, or elite). The goal of testing is to establish an athletic profile for each athlete—a set of scores that can be used as a starting point and reevaluated throughout the season to measure improvement of each athlete. So use the scores to chart the progression of each member of the team as well as the team totals.

Once the testing is complete, look up the results on the tables to determine the point value for each performance. The values are based on a mean score derived from the test results of many athletes of many abilities. Thus, if you are a high school player,

Table 2.2   Sample Team Testing Database

								Smith Volleyball
Test >>	No-step VL (in)*	One-step VL (in)*	Pts	Three-hop (ft, in)	Pts	20-yd sprint (sec)	Pts
Sarah Jones	17.0	18.5	7	19'6"	6	3.39	4
Jane Smith	22.0	21.0	8	22'1"	8	3.25	6
Lindsey Alba	18.5	20.5	8	18'9"	6	3.47	4
Missy Lane	19.0	19.0	7	19'6"	6	3.26	5
Kim White	15.5	16.5	5	19'2"	6	3.48	4
Kathy Smith	18.0	19.5	7	20'9"	7	3.42	4
Ann Williams	18.0	18.5	7	18'3"	5	3.65	3
Donna Phils	17.0	18.0	6	16'7"	4	3.58	3
Team average	18.1	19.0	7	19'4"	6	3.44	4
HS average	16.0	17.0	6	18'6"	6	3.25	6

*For the no-step and one-step vertical leap tests, use the lowest points score from the two tests.
1 inch = 2.54 centimeters; 1 foot = 0.3048 meters; 1 yard = 0.9144 meters.

you wouldn't expect to test as high as an elite athlete in your sport. Use the following guidelines to get an idea of what types of results to expect and to guide you in picking goal scores.

High school junior varsity: five points
High school varsity: six points
College: seven to eight points
Elite (professional or Olympic): nine to ten points

If you are a coach and you have picked out the specific tests you would like to use for your team (see table 2.1 for help), you can save your data in a spreadsheet program like Microsoft® Excel and create team databases (see table 2.2 for an example).

Notice how precise and objective this system is. The horizontal row represents the individual athlete's raw scores and point designation for each test. The column to the far right represents the athlete's total score (point value). We like to refer to this as the athleticism profile score. The raw scores in each vertical column are averaged for each test. The last space in the vertical column represents the average score for high school athletes. Coaches can use this profile in several ways.

- To evaluate an athlete's current level of athleticism
- To evaluate an athlete's overall improvement after a training program
- To compare athletes' relative strengths and weaknesses within a team
- To compare individual and team results to national averages
- To determine an athlete's strength and weaknesses for future development

Table 2.3 provides a team profile chart and table 2.4 (page 24) provides an individual profile chart that you can copy and use to record your own team's testing data.

T-test (sec)	Pts	300-yd shuttle (sec)	Pts	Push-up (reps)	Pts	Sit-up (reps)	Pts	Sit-and-reach (in)	Pts	Total points
10.74	3	67.0	6	24	8	55	10	3	6	50
9.99	6	64.5	7	28	9	53	9	2	5	58
10.20	5	67.0	6	32	10	52	9	2	5	53
9.40	8	66.5	6	17	5	35	6	5	7	50
10.03	5	68.5	5	37	10	32	5	7	8	48
10.46	4	68.0	5	17	5	20	3	4	6	41
10.88	2	67.5	6	35	10	30	5	8	8	46
10.60	3	70.0	4	19	6	35	6	-1	3	35
10.29	4	67.37	6	26	8	39	6	3.75	6	47
10.00	6	67.0	6	20	6	39	6	4	6	48

Table 2.3 Team Testing Profile Chart

Test >> Player name	Player pos.	Grade	Height	Test name	Pts	Test name	Pts	Test name	Pts	Test name	Pts
Team average											

From *Athletic Strength for Women* by David Oliver and Dana Healy, 2005, Champaign, IL: Human Kinetics.

Test name		Test name		Test name		Test name		Test name		Test name		Total points
	Pts		Pts		Pts		Pts		Pts		Pts	

Table 2.4 Individual Testing Profile Chart

Choose your individual tests from this chart and perform them in this order.

Name								
	Test 1 date		Test 2 date		Test 3 date		Test 4 date	
Test	Score	Points	Score	Points	Score	Points	Score	Points
No-step vertical leap								
One-step vertical leap								
Three-hop test								
Broad-jump test								
20-yd sprint								
40-yd sprint								
20-yd shuttle								
T-test								
300-yd shuttle								
Leger beep test								
Mile run								
Push-up test								
Pull-up test								
Sit-up test								
Sit-and-reach test								

Note: The last several rows are for sport-specific testing. Perform other specific strength or power testing such as bench press, squat, and power clean under strict supervision by your strength and conditioning coach.

From *Athletic Strength for Women* by David Oliver and Dana Healy, 2005, Champaign, IL: Human Kinetics.

NO-STEP VERTICAL LEAP

This test measures pure leg and hip power. The no-step vertical leap may be performed using a Vertec (available at most commercial gyms, schools, or testing facilities) or jump mat (which measures the jump electronically), or performed against a wall.

Raw score (in)	Points
≥21.5	10
20.0-21.4	9
18.5-19.9	8
17.0-18.4	7
16.0-16.9	6
14.5-15.9	5
13.0-14.4	4
12.0-12.9	3
11.0-11.9	2
≤10.9	1

1 inch = 2.54 centimeters

1. Stand next to the wall, feet parallel to one another and to the wall. Reach up the wall with your arm extended while a coach measures where your fingertips reach on the wall.

2. Explode upward extending your arms overhead, and touch the highest mark you can on the Vertec or wall.

3. Obtain the final measurement by taking the total jump height minus the standing height. For example, if your total jump height is 110 inches and standing reach height is 89 inches, you have a 21-inch no-step vertical leap.

4. Compare your score to those in the raw-score column of the table shown on this page.

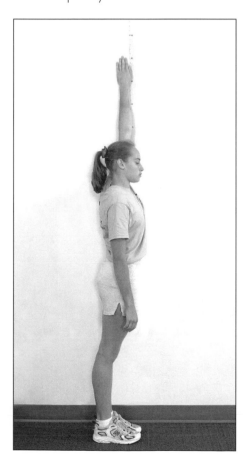
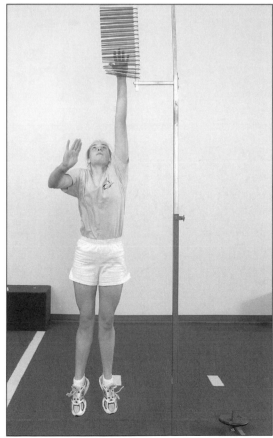

ONE-STEP VERTICAL LEAP

This test measures leg power and the ability to transfer horizontal momentum to vertical power.

1. Stand next to the wall, feet parallel to one another and to the wall. Reach up the wall with your arm extended while a coach measures where your fingertips reach on the wall.

2. Position yourself one step away from your takeoff point.

3. From this position take one gather step, and jump vertically with a maximal effort.

4. Obtain the final measurement by taking the total jump height minus the standing height and compare to your score for the no-step vertical leap.

Raw score (in)	Points
≥23.0	10
21.5-22.9	9
20.0-21.4	8
18.5-19.9	7
17.0-18.4	6
15.5-16.9	5
14.0-15.4	4
13.0-13.9	3
12.0-12.9	2
≤11.9	1

1 inch = 2.54 centimeters

Note that volleyball players should use a two-step volleyball approach and a gather followed by takeoff. Volleyball coaches then measure the total jump height rather than the total jump height minus standing reach.

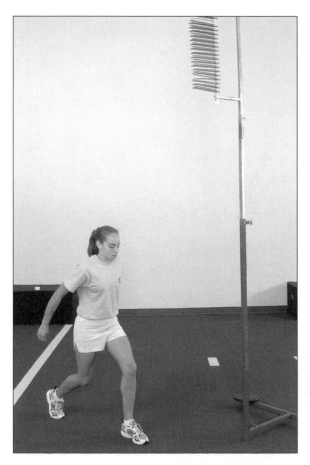

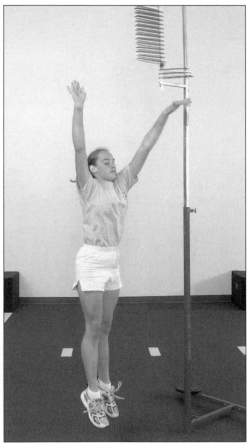

THREE-HOP TEST

This test measures lower-extremity power and balance. Set up the test by extending a tape measure on the floor or ground about 30 feet.

1. Position yourself at one end of the measuring tape.

2. When set, explode off the line, pushing with both legs. Upon landing complete two more hops.

3. Maintain continuous movement throughout the test. If you stop at any point between the takeoff and the final landing, the jump does not count, and you must retest. The distance is measured at the back of the heel after the final hop.

Raw score (ft, in)	Points
≥24'6"	10
23'0"-24'5"	9
21'6"-22'11"	8
20'0"-21'5"	7
18'6"-19'11"	6
17'0"-18'5"	5
15'6"-16'11"	4
14'0"-15'5"	3
13'0"-13'11"	2
≤12'11"	1

1 inch = 2.54 centimeters; 1 foot = 0.3048 meters

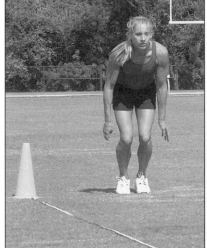

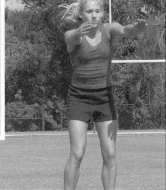

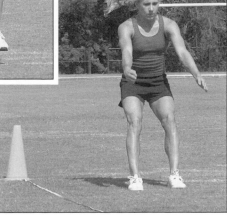

BROAD-JUMP TEST

The broad jump measures explosive power of the lower extremity. It differs from the three-hop test because it removes the transition between the jumps and takes out the balance and timing elements. Sports like swimming and diving might test the broad jump to evaluate explosiveness off the blocks or platform. Set up the test by extending a tape measure on the floor about eight feet.

1. Position yourself at one end of the measuring tape.
2. When set, explode off the line, pushing with both legs.
3. Measure the end of the jump from the back of the heel. If the you fall back, the test does not count, and you must retest.

Raw score (ft, in)	Points
≥7'0"	10
6'8"-6'11"	9
6'4"-6'7"	8
6'0"-6'3"	7
5'8"-5'11"	6
5'4"-5'7"	5
5'0"-5'3"	4
4'8"-4'11"	3
4'4"-4'7"	2
≤4'3"	1

1 inch = 2.54 centimeters; 1 foot = 0.3048 meters

20-YARD SPRINT

This test measures acceleration.

1. Mark a start and a finish line 20 yards apart on a court or playing field. Place the timer at the finish line.
2. Using a standing start or a three-point start (with one hand down), sprint from the start line to the finish line.
3. The timer should start the watch on your first movement and stop the watch as the chest breaks the plane of the finish line.

Raw score (sec)	Points
≤3.00	10
3.01-3.05	9
3.06-3.10	8
3.11-3.15	7
3.16-3.25	6
3.26-3.35	5
3.36-3.50	4
3.51-3.70	3
3.71-3.80	2
≥3.81	1

1 yard = 0.9144 meters

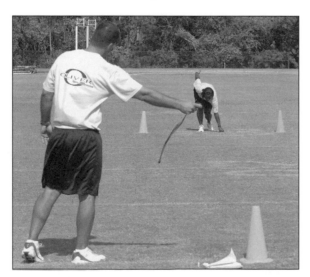

40-YARD SPRINT

This test measures acceleration and speed.

1. Measure a distance of 40 yards on a field and have the timer stand at the finish line.

2. Perform the 40 the same way as the 20-yard sprint. The timer starts the watch on your first movement.

Raw score (sec)	Points
≤5.0	10
5.1-5.2	9
5.3-5.4	8
5.5-5.6	7
5.7-5.8	6
5.9-6.0	5
6.1-6.2	4
6.3-6.4	3
6.5-6.6	2
≥6.7	1

1 yard = 0.9144 meters

20-YARD SHUTTLE

This test measures lateral speed and lateral acceleration and deceleration (agility).

1. Use a court or a field with a flat running surface, and set up three cones five yards apart from each other in a straight line. Near the end cones mark a short line perpendicular to the straight line formed by the cones. This line will provide a target for the athlete to touch.

2. Straddle the middle cone while facing it and place one hand on the ground.

3. Sprint from the start position to the end cone on the right.

4. Touch the short line near the cone while making a right-footed cut, change direction, and run past the middle cone to the other end cone.

Raw score (sec)	Points
≤4.2	10
4.3-4.4	9
4.5-4.6	8
4.7-4.8	7
4.9-5.0	6
5.1-5.2	5
5.3-5.4	4
5.5-5.6	3
5.7-5.8	2
≥5.9	1

1 yard = 0.9144 meters

5. Touch the line near the cone, cutting off the left foot, and finish by running past the middle cone. In doing so you will have completed a right-footed cut and a left-footed cut.

6. Perform the test starting with a right-footed cut and then again starting with a left cut. This way you will measure cutting speed in both directions to evaluate weaknesses.

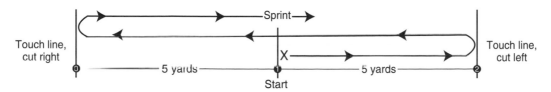

T-TEST

This test measures forward, lateral, and backward agility.

1. Set up the test by measuring two 10-yard lines to form a T. Place cone 1 at the base of the T and cone 2 at the other end of the vertical line, where the two lines meet. Place cone three on the right end of the horizontal line and cone four on the left end. The start-finish line is at cone 1.

2. Sprint forward from cone one to cone 2.

3. Run just past cone 2, and shuffle right to cone 3.

4. Plant the right foot, turn, and sprint to cone 4.

5. Change direction at cone 4, and shuffle right to cone 2.

6. At cone 2, backpedal to the start-finish line. The timer starts the clock on the first movement and stops the clock when the back crosses the line.

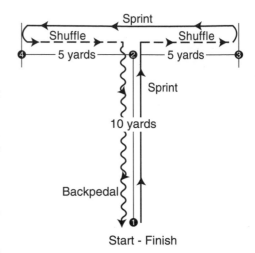

Start - Finish

Raw score (sec)	Points
≤9.00	10
9.01-9.25	9
9.26-9.50	8
9.51-9.75	7
9.76-10.00	6
10.01-10.25	5
10.26-10.50	4
10.51-10.80	3
10.81-11.10	2
≥11.11	1

1 yard = 0.9144 meters

LEGER BEEP TEST

This test measures cardiovascular endurance. These aerobic endurance tests are more specific to sport than other endurance tests because they involve increasing rates of speed and changes of direction. The athlete must successfully cover the 20-meter course at the slower speeds before moving on to the next, quicker rates as determined by the interval between two beeps played on a cassette. The starting speed of most beep tests is 8 to 8.5 kilometers (5 to 5.28 miles) per hour, and each minute the speed is increased .5 kilometers (.62 miles) per hour by decreasing the interval between beeps. The Leger test we present is a continuous version.

Tapes and CDs for the Leger beep test are available for purchase from many national coaching associations. Another similar beep test was developed by Jens Bangsbo.

Raw score— Leger (stages)	Raw score— Bangsbo (stages)	Points
12	13	10
11	12	9
10	11	8
9	10	7
8	9	6
7	8	5
6	7	4
5	6	3
4	5	2
3	4	1

1. Set up the test by marking off a lane 20 meters long. You can use cones or lines to mark off each end of the lane.

2. Start at one end of the lane, facing the cone or mark at the other end.

3. Start each leg (trip down the lane) when the audio tape beeps, and try to reach the end of the lane and pivot at the line at the moment the next beep sounds (not quicker or slower). A single beep indicates the completion of the previous interval and the start of the next interval.

4. The test ends when the you are unable to get within three meters of the line before the beep for two consecutive times.

5. Use the scoring table to determine your score. Each raw score indicates the number of minutes (often noted as stages on the tape) you were able to complete.

300-YARD SHUTTLE

This test measures lactate threshold. Lactate threshold is important for measuring an athlete's game readiness. The ability to recover over repetitive intervals of running is the best measure of game fitness. When athletes produce lactic acid in the muscles, performance may be diminished significantly if they are unable to recover quickly. This test is best for sports like basketball, field hockey, soccer, and others that require similar energy needs. This is one of our favorite tests.

1. Place two cones 25 yards apart. Mark a short line perpendicular to the straight line formed by the cones near each cone.

2. Sprint six complete trips (from cone one to cone 2 and back to cone 1 equals one trip) for a distance of 300 yards. Touch the foot to the short line at each end of the 25 yards. The test begins on the timer's command and ends when you pass the start-finish line.

Raw score (sec) Average of two trials	Points
≤59.9	10
60.0-61.9	9
62.0-63.9	8
64.0-65.9	7
66.0-67.9	6
68.0-69.9	5
70.0-71.9	4
72.0-73.9	3
74.0-75.9	2
≥76.0	1

1 yard = 0.9144 meters

You will have 5 minutes to recover before starting the second trial. Your score is the average of the two trials. For example, if you complete trial one in 65 seconds and trial two in 67 seconds, your score is 66 seconds. A coach can use the difference between trials as an indicator of fitness. For instance, athletes who are in game condition usually will score on the second trial within 1 to 2 seconds of the first trial. A difference of 4 seconds suggests that the athlete does not clear lactate from her system efficiently. Interval training sessions are the best way to enhance your lactate threshold and increase your rate of recovery.

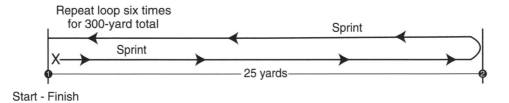

Repeat loop six times
for 300-yard total

Sprint

Sprint

X

25 yards

1

2

Start - Finish

MILE RUN

This test measures cardiovascular strength—the athlete's ability to use oxygen for energy. Perform this test on a standard 400-meter track.

1. Run one mile on a measured course or track.
2. Compare your finish time with the standards in the table.

Raw score (min:sec)	Points
≤6:29	10
6:30-7:14	9
7:15-7:59	8
8:00-8:44	7
8:45-9:29	6
9:30-10:14	5
10:15-10:59	4
11:00-11:44	3
11:45-12:29	2
≥12:30	1

1 mile = 1.609 kilometers

Based on Cooper Institute's Physical Fitness Norms for Law Enforcement, the Presidential Physical Fitness Award Program, and national physical fitness standards.

PULL-UP TEST

The pull-up measures upper-extremity strength and endurance. School-age girls typically perform an arm-hang instead. However, as those young women become stronger through strength training, they should add this test to their profile. Pull-ups test strength in the upper-extremity pulling muscles (latissimus dorsi, biceps, and wrist flexors).

1. Grip the bar with palms facing toward the body.
2. Start from a fully extended position with straight elbows.
3. Pull up until the chin passes the bar. Repeat to failure

Raw score (reps)	Points
≥10	10
9	9
8	8
7	7
6	6
5	5
4	4
3	3
2	2
1	1

PUSH-UP TEST

This test measures upper-body strength and endurance.

1. Place a pad below the chest at a height that allows a 90-degree angle at the elbow when in the down position.
2. During each repetition maintain a straight body position.
3. Complete as many repetitions as possible in 60 seconds. You will rest in the up position. If the knee touches the ground during rest, the test is over. Do not count repetitions that do not achieve the 90-degree angle.

Raw score (reps)	Points
≥30	10
27-29	9
24-26	8
21-23	7
18-20	6
15-17	5
12-14	4
9-11	3
7-8	2
≤6	1

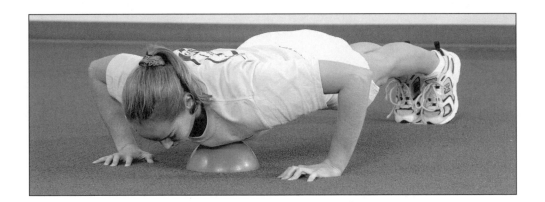

SIT-UP TEST

This test measures abdominal muscle endurance.

1. Start on the back with knees bent and arms crossed with hands on the shoulders. A partner will hold the feet and count repetitions for 60 seconds.

2. Curl up so that the elbows touch the knees. The repetition is completed by curling down so that the low back touches the ground. Repetitions are not counted if the hands leave the shoulders, if the elbows do not touch the knees, or if the low back does not touch the ground.

Raw score (reps)	Points
≥55	10
50-54	9
45-49	8
40-44	7
35-39	6
30-34	5
25-29	4
20-24	3
16-19	2
≤15	1

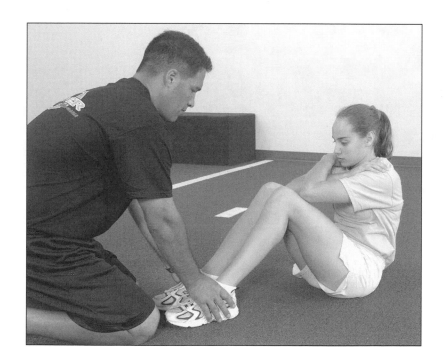

SIT-AND-REACH TEST

This test measures hamstring flexibility. Lack of hamstring flexibility is the primary contributor to low back problems in athletes. It can also contribute to decreased speed and agility and expose athletes to muscle strains.

1. Use a sit-and-reach box or a tape measure and 12-inch-high box.
2. Sit with bare feet flat against the box.
3. Reach forward as far as you can with palms on the box and the knees flat on the floor. Move in and out of the stretch slowly.
4. Perform three trials, holding each stretch for 2 seconds. Measure the distance past your feet that you are able to reach to determine your raw score.

Raw score (in)	Points
≥12	10
+10 or +11	9
+8 or +7	8
+6 or +5	7
+4 or +3	6
+2 or +1	5
0	4
-2 or -1	3
-4 or -3	2
≤-5	1

1 inch = 2.54 centimeters

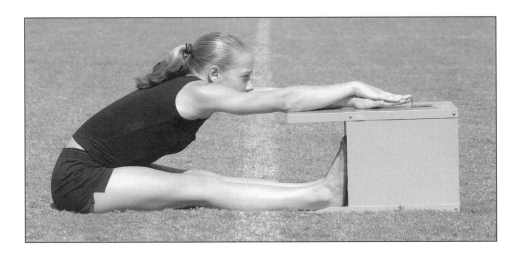

Coaches often refer to their teams or individual athletes as fast, strong, or quick without always knowing how fast, how strong, or how quick. Testing a team requires extra work for coaches, but the data obtained is invaluable. The coach will use this data to set goals for each athlete and for the team. Testing data also helps coaches gauge individual growth over time, and is useful in determining whether the team's strength and conditioning program is working. Ultimately the test results allow the coach to objectively quantify the exact strength, speed, and power gains made by their athletes. Testing gives you a solid baseline as you begin your strength and conditioning program.

Part II

Getting Stronger

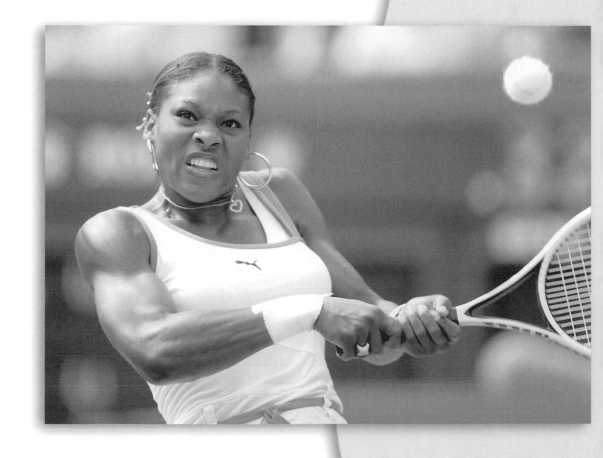

3

Shoulder Support

In many sports the muscles of the shoulder play a major role in primary movements and in the stabilization of the joint during the performance of a sport skill. For example, the latissimus dorsi muscles of the upper back give a swimmer her power for the breaststroke. The supraspinatus muscle of the rotator cuff group is responsible for deceleration of the arm after a spike in volleyball and is a major contributor to keeping the shoulder free of injury. It is crucial that athletes perform exercises that strengthen these muscles, creating a stable joint that reduces the chance for injury and that improves performance. In this chapter we present an anatomical look at the shoulder joint and its primary function in sport. We also provide insight into current trends in injuries to the female athlete's shoulder and provide specific exercises for protecting this sophisticated joint.

Consider your body as one kinetic chain—moving one part of the body depends on other parts of the body, and power generated by large muscle groups is transferred to other muscle groups. Your body is linked from your feet to the tips of your fingers. The power generated in your legs is transferred through your hips, torso, shoulders, and arms and finally reaches your hands. Weakness in any part of the chain contributes to a loss of power. The shoulder joint is the last *major* link in the chain. Weakness in the shoulder therefore reduces your ability to perform many movements optimally and exposes you to a greater risk of injury. An aggressive upper-body strength and power program is essential for your overall performance. We detail this type of program in this chapter.

STRUCTURE OF THE SHOULDER

Two primary components make up all joints. *Bones* provide the basic structure and support for joints. *Soft tissue* is composed of muscles, tendons, ligaments, and cartilage. Soft tissue works to move bones through ranges of motion while also providing support and shock absorption.

The shoulder joint complex is made up of three primary bones. The scapula, clavicle, and humerus bones provide the primary structure and areas of attachment for the muscles of the shoulder (see figures 3.1*a* and *b*). The *scapula*, often called the shoulder blade, provides a primary attachment for many muscles on the posterior (back) aspect of the shoulder. The rotator cuff muscle group's primary attachments are on the scapula. The scapula makes up part of the glenohumeral (GH) joint (the primary ball and socket). This is the primary joint around which all movement revolves. The *clavicle*, commonly referred to as the collarbone, is a small s-shaped bone located at the anterior (front) part of the shoulder complex, and it is a part of two specific joints, the acromioclavicular (AC) and the sternoclavicular (SC). The acromioclavicular joint is a primary location for injury in sport. Lacrosse, field hockey, and ice hockey involve

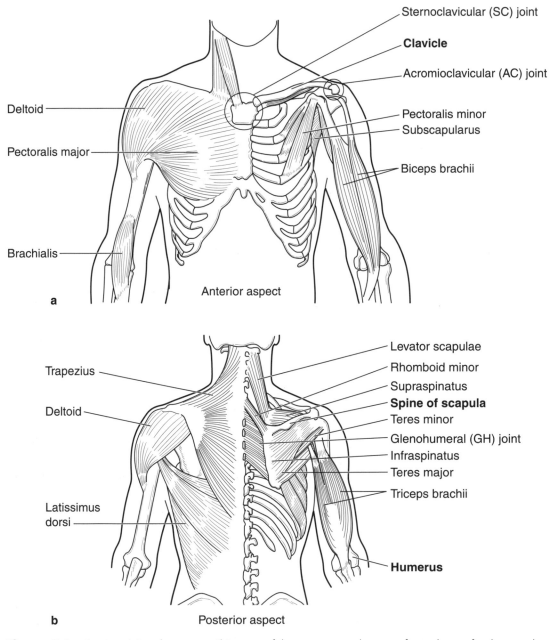

Figure 3.1 Anterior *(a)* and posterior *(b)* views of the structure and areas of attachment for the muscles of the shoulder complex.

Reprinted, by permission, from J. Loudon, S. Bell, J. Johnston, 1998, *The clinical orthopedic assessment guide* (Champaign, IL: Human Kinetics), 87.

heavy contact with other players or frequent contact with the ground. Contact between the shoulder and the ground or falling with an outstretched arm can cause an AC joint separation injury. The *humerus* is the bone of the upper arm. It provides the insertion for the rotator cuff muscle group and is responsible for all dynamic movement around the shoulder joint.

At least nine major muscles make up the shoulder complex. Muscles contract and relax around a joint to create movement but also act as secondary stabilizers of the joint. Illustrated in figures 3.1*a* and *b* are the major muscles that attach to the bones of the shoulder. These muscles can be separated into three areas: rotator cuff muscles, which are primarily responsible for rotation of the upper arm; anterior muscles, which raise and lower the upper arm and in some cases help rotate it; and posterior muscles, which also raise, lower, and rotate the upper arm and shoulder (see table 3.1).

The shoulder joint complex is made up of four primary joints held together by ligaments. A ligament attaches bone to bone and acts as the primary stabilizer of the joint. Ligaments provide joints a significant source of strength, but when they are injured, the joint loses its stability to varying degrees. Ligaments are inflexible, taut, and are usually short and thick. Think of a ligament as a climbing rope, which has a small amount of give but a solid end point. These characteristics make ligaments difficult to injure, but if torn, the injury can cause major joint problems. Ligaments heal slowly because of their poor blood supply. Athletes who maintain strong secondary support to their joints through strong, balanced muscles are more likely to maintain healthy joints.

Notice in figure 3.1*a* that the **sternoclavicular (SC) joint** connects the sternum to the clavicle. This joint serves as the axis of movement at the sternum when elevating the shoulder. It links the shoulder to the chest. The **acromioclavicular (AC) joint** is a primary area of stabilization and attachment for muscles of the shoulder joint. Injuries to the AC ligament cause instability and laxity around the shoulder joint complex. The acromion is a focal bony structure and area for muscle and tendon attachment. Injury and laxity at the AC joint affect the function of the rotator cuff muscle group. The **glenohumeral (GH) joint** is the region of insertion for the humerus on the glenoid fossa

Table 3.1 Muscles of the Shoulder Complex and Their Functions

Group	Muscle	Primary function
Rotator cuff	Supraspinatus	External rotation of the humerus
	Infraspinatus Teres minor Subscapularus	Internal rotation of the humerus
Anterior	Pectoralis major and minor	Internal rotation of the humerus
	Deltoid	Elevation of the humerus
Posterior	Latissimus dorsi Teres major	Internal rotation of the humerus
	Deltoid	Elevation of the humerus
	Trapezius	Elevation of the scapula

of the scapula. It is the primary ball-and-socket joint of the shoulder complex. Injuries to this joint are usually dislocations and are associated with contact but can occur if the anterior part of the shoulder is lax. The fourth joint of the shoulder complex (not pictured) is the **coracoclavicular joint**.

SHOULDERS AT WORK

The muscles of the shoulder joint function in two primary ways.

1. They function as *prime movers*. That is, they work through a given range of motion (ROM) to cause the movement.
2. They also function as *stabilizers*. A muscle that stabilizes a joint contracts isometrically (does not move through a range of motion) and protects the joint during exercise and competition.

A swimmer performing freestyle (front crawl) uses her latissimus dorsi as a prime mover for pulling and serratus to stabilize her scapula during the pull. In sports where throwing, striking, or physical defensive play is involved, female athletes benefit from strength and power training programs as much as their male counterparts do. Increasing muscle strength around the shoulder joint enhances an athlete's ability to throw with greater velocity and defend with more confidence because she is now more likely to dominate her opponent. With this increased strength and power also comes the need for an increased ability to protect the joint from injury. If an athlete throws a softball with greater velocity, she must also gain the corresponding ability to decelerate her arm using the supraspinatus muscle of the rotator cuff.

In the figure at the left you can see the importance of the shoulder's prime movers when performing a movement like a spike in volleyball. The muscles around the shoulder joint act as prime movers and stabilizers.

Athletes or coaches who want to evaluate upper-body strength and stability of the shoulder joint can perform general strength testing (see chapter 2) and should consult their team athletic trainer, strength and conditioning coach, or physician for more specific manual muscle testing.

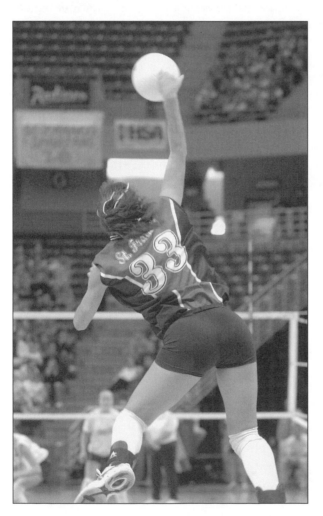

Properly trained pectoralis, latissimus dorsi, and rotatotor cuff muscle groups provide both the range of motion and the joint protection required to execute a powerful spike.

Several common injuries can occur in the shoulder joint if athletes fail to properly strengthen them. Some of the most common injuries include the following:

Overuse injuries are associated with repetitive bouts of trauma to a specific joint. These injuries are usually chronic, that is they occur and then recur over increasing periods of time. Tendinitis, bursitis, and capsulitis are examples of overuse injuries—an "itis" of any kind is associated with inflammation to soft tissue at the joint. Gymnasts often suffer from biceps tendinitis or bursitis of the shoulder due to repetitive bouts of pulling movements. A softball pitcher or swimmer may see similar problems. Proper strengthening of the muscles at the joint involved and adequate resting of the affected area after training or competition prevent overuse injuries.

Sprains are associated with injury to a ligament. As acute trauma injuries, they occur instantaneously. There are three different degrees of sprains. First-degree sprains are most common and involve partial tearing of the ligament, whereas third-degree sprains involve a complete tearing or rupture of the ligament. Second-degree sprains fall somewhere in between. Ruptured ligaments often require surgery because of their lack of blood flow and poor healing capabilities. A first-degree sprain of an AC joint may occur when a field hockey player is knocked to the ground and lands on the anterior aspect of her shoulder joint. The fall causes a partial separation of the AC joint. AC separations are often slow healing, and they require strengthening of the support muscles around the joint.

Strains are another acute injury common to athletes. Shoulder muscle strains often occur to the rotator cuff muscles. Athletes who throw and strike strain the supraspinatus muscle primarily. Muscle strains are more easily managed than sprains because of the rich supply of blood to the muscle. Strains can usually be treated with RICE (rest, ice, compress, and elevate); however, as with any injury, it is always best to check with an athletic trainer or physician before you treat yourself.

Dislocations of the shoulder are serious acute trauma injuries and require immediate medical attention. Never try to "pop back" your shoulder if it is dislocated. Other injuries may have occurred with the dislocation, and it would be dangerous to try to manipulate it yourself. Dislocations occur at the GH joint and involve displacement of the ball and socket. These injuries are usually associated with body contact, falling on an outstretched hand, vaulting in gymnastics, and other movements that cause forceful impact on the joint.

Increasing your overall strength not only gives you a better chance to maintain the stability of the joint and increase your overall power, but may also help to protect the joint against injuries like those just presented.

INCREASING SHOULDER STRENGTH AND STABILITY

This chapter is devoted to helping you understand the anatomy and function of the shoulder joint. Whether you are a coach or an athlete, a firm understanding of the body will help you determine the appropriate training method for improving performance and reducing the risk of injury.

In chapter 7 we provide explosive exercises that involve much larger muscle groups that work with the shoulder complex (chest and back). The exercises in this chapter, however, are specific to the rotator cuff muscle group and specific muscles around the shoulder joint and focus on developing strength and joint stability. This series of exercises is appropriate for athletes of all age groups.

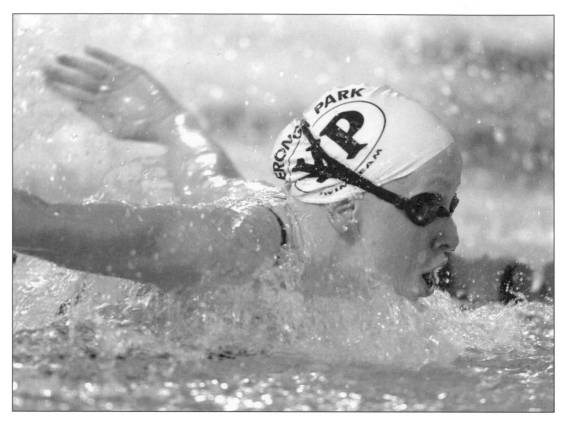

Swimmers use their rotator cuff musculature to perform many strokes, but they especially rely on it to swim the butterfly.

DUMBBELL ROTATOR CUFF ROUTINE

This routine builds a solid base of strength and muscular endurance. It can also be used during the in-season for most sports because it promotes new blood flow, which helps remove the toxins and waste that have built up in the muscles during training. It is an excellent way to maintain strength and to promote healthy shoulder joints during the competitive season. This routine is great for athletes in all sports but should be common practice for golfers, volleyball players, swimmers, and softball players—those who participate in sports that rely on the rotator cuff for many of their movements.

Perform this routine in sequence, three or four times a week. Perform 12 repetitions of each exercise with 3- to 5-pound (1.5- to 2-kilogram) dumbbells. Rest 10 seconds after each exercise before going on to the next one.

45-DEGREE SHOULDER FLEXION

This exercise works the supraspinatus (external rotator) and posterior deltoid muscles.

1. Stand with knees slightly bent and arms straight and positioned at the hips with thumbs down.
2. Slowly raise the dumbbells up and away from the body at a 45-degree angle without using the trapezius muscles to raise the arms. Make sure that the shoulders stay neutral and don't rise up toward the ears.
3. Stop at shoulder height and hold for 1 second before lowering slowly.

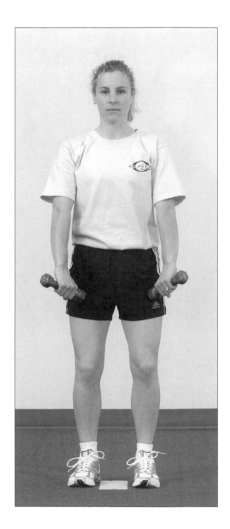
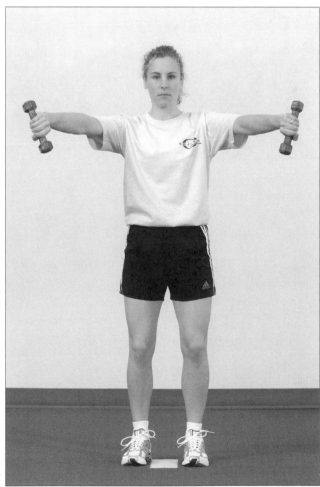

FRONT RAISE

This exercise works the anterior deltoid muscles.

1. Stand with knees slightly bent, and arms straight at the side with thumbs up.
2. Slowly raise the dumbbells in front of you, keeping the arms straight until the hands reach shoulder height.
3. Hold for 1 second at the top of the movement before lowering slowly.

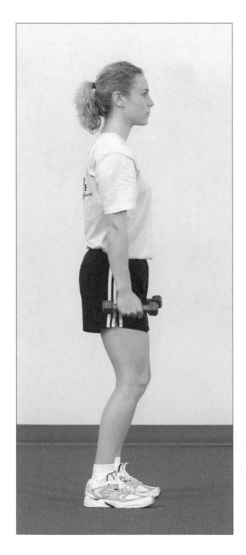 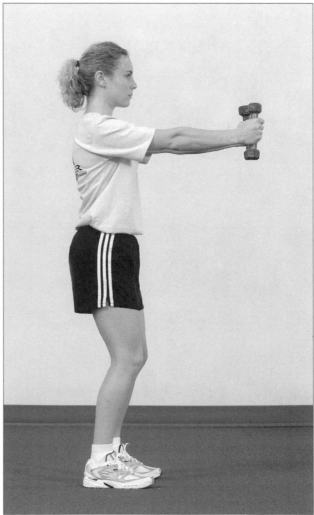

LATERAL RAISE

This exercise works the deltoids and trapezius muscles.

1. Stand with knees slightly bent and elbows bent at 90 degrees. Position elbows at the side with thumbs up.
2. Keeping the elbows bent, slowly raise the dumbbells up and out until they reach shoulder height.
3. Hold for 1 second at the top of the movement before lowering slowly.

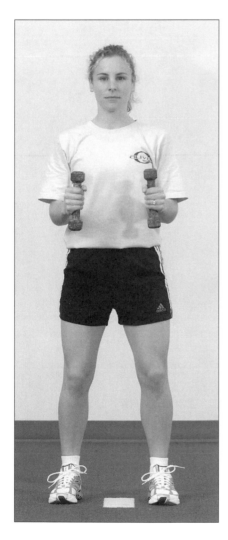
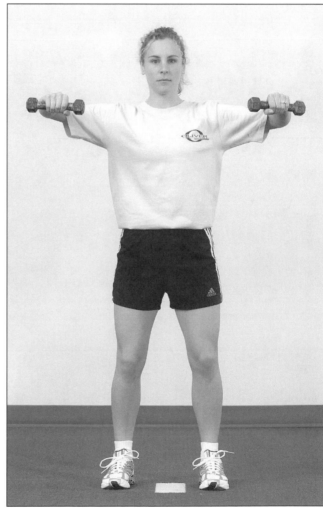

OVERHEAD SIDE RAISE

This exercise works the anterior deltoid muscles.

1. Stand with the knees slightly bent.
2. Start with the dumbbells touching at hip level and palms facing forward.
3. Slowly raise the dumbbells laterally out to the side, bending the arms slightly. Move the dumbbells up past the shoulder until they touch over the head.
4. Hold for 1 second at the top of the movement before lowering slowly.

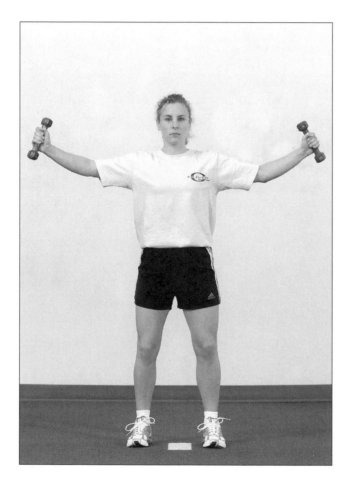
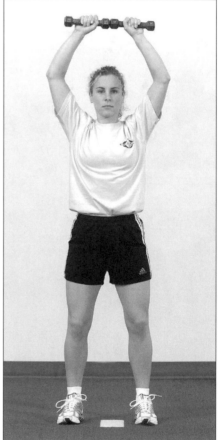

EXTERNAL ROTATION

This exercise works the supraspinatus muscle.

1. Stand with knees slightly bent.
2. Bend elbows at 90 degrees, keeping upper arms parallel to the ground and lower arms hanging down with dumbbells at waist-level.
3. Rotate the dumbbells 180 degrees so that they are now at head height.
4. Hold for 1 second at the top of the movement before lowering slowly.

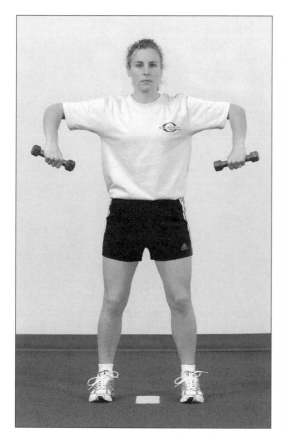
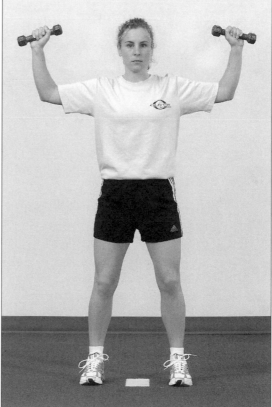

DIAGONAL RAISE

This exercise works the muscles of the rotator cuff and the deltoids.

1. Stand with knees slightly bent.
2. Start with one hand at the opposite hip, palm facing in and the thumb out.
3. Raise the dumbbell up and away diagonally at a 45-degree angle until it is over the opposite shoulder with the thumb pointing behind you.
4. Hold for 1 second at the top of the movement before slowly lowering the dumbbell.
5. Repeat on each side.

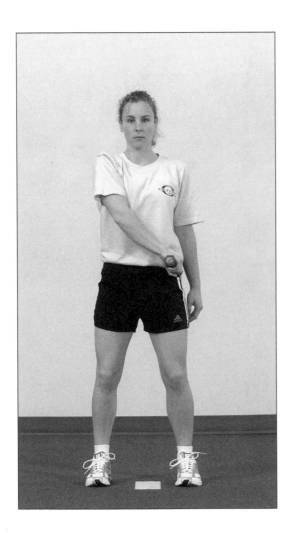
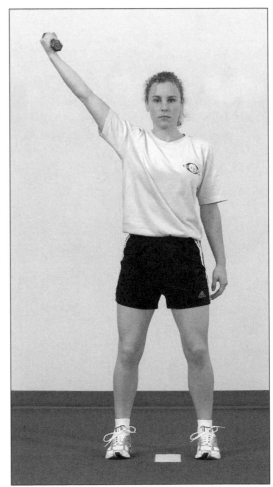

INTERNAL ROTATION

This exercise works the muscles of the rotator cuff and the subscapularus. For this exercise only you may use more than 5 pounds (2 kilograms).

1. Lie faceup on a bench or exercise table. Bend the knees.
2. Position the arm against the side of the body with the elbow bent at 90 degrees and the palm facing up.
3. Slowly raise the dumbbell upward so that the forearm finishes in a position perpendicular to the table.
4. Hold for 1 second at the top of the movement before slowly lowering the dumbbell.

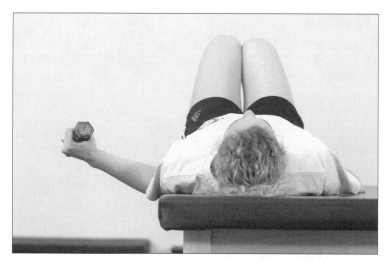

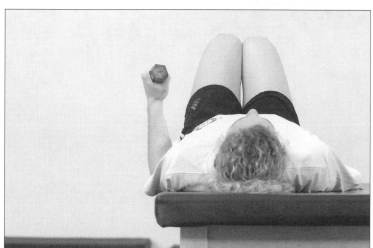

BODY-WEIGHT SHOULDER STABILIZATION ROUTINE

The body-weight routine is a safe and effective way for an athlete to stabilize the shoulder in a functional way. Functional training incorporates a series of multijoint exercises that more directly simulate the movements used in sport. This routine is excellent for preventing injuries to the shoulder girdle while also promoting low back and abdominal strength. Because these exercises work the core as well as the shoulder, they are appropriate for athletes of most sports. Perform this routine in sequence.

FOREARM PUSH-UP

The exercise works the scapular stabilizers, serratus, and abdominal muscles.

1. Lie facedown on the floor.
2. Assume a straight body position while propping yourself up on the forearms. A partner can offer resistance as shown in the photo.
3. Concentrate on keeping the muscles of the shoulder girdle and trunk contracted as you hold this position for 30 seconds.
4. Repeat the exercise twice, progressing to 1 minute.

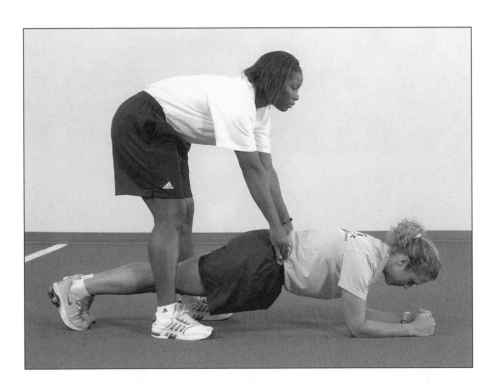

FOREARM SIDE RAISE

The exercise works the scapular stabilizers, serratus, and abdominal muscles.

1. Lie on your side on the floor.
2. Assume a straight body, side-lying position while propping yourself up on one forearm. Your body should form a 30- to 45-degree angle with the ground.
3. A partner provides resistance by placing her hands on your side.
4. Concentrate on keeping the muscles of the shoulder girdle and trunk contracted to push against the resistance.
5. Hold the position for 30 seconds.
6. Repeat twice on each side, progressing to 1 minute.

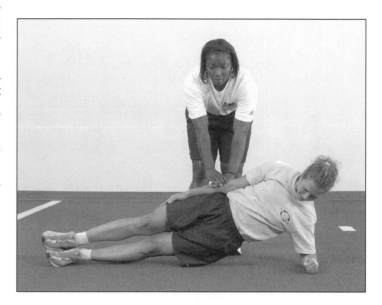

BACK RAISE

The exercise works the scapular stabilizers, serratus, and abdominal muscles.

1. Lie faceup on the floor.
2. Assume a straight body, back-lying position while propping yourself up on the forearms.
3. A partner provides resistance by placing her hands on your hips. Raise up against your partner's resistance.
4. Concentrate on keeping the muscles of the shoulder girdle and trunk contracted while you hold the position for 30 seconds.
5. Repeat it twice, progressing to 1 minute.

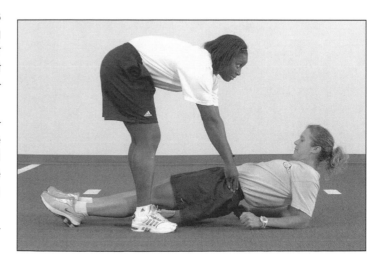

BOX WALK

This exercise works the pectoralis, triceps, scapular stabilizers, and serratus.

1. Form an arc with three or four boxes set 24 inches (60 centimeters) apart. The boxes should be four to six inches high.
2. Start at one side of the boxes in a push-up position.
3. Raise the arm closest to the box first to "walk" the hands on top of the first box.
4. Once both hands are on top of the first box, step them off the box to the floor and move to the second box the same way.
5. Complete a full trip of the box set and return for one complete repetition.
6. Perform two or three sets of two trips over all the boxes and back.
7. Make sure to keep the body in a stable position throughout the movement.
8. Start with 4-inch boxes and work up to 6 inches (10 to 15 centimeters).

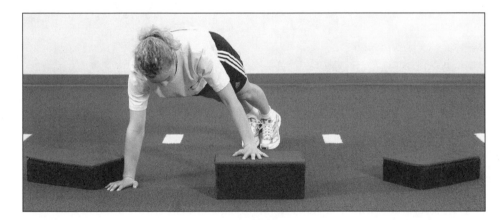

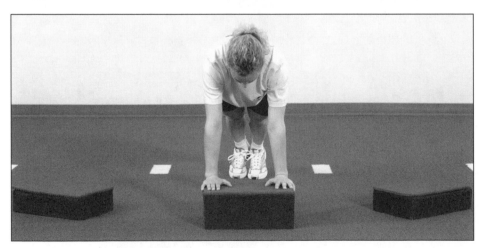

OTHER UPPER-EXTREMITY STRENGTHENERS

You are probably already familiar with and have performed many of the exercises in this next group. For this reason, we do not include photos.

BENCH PRESS

This exercise primarily works the pectoralis (chest) and triceps muscles and develops chest strength for sports movements that involve pushing, shooting, and passing. You can perform this exercise using a barbell or using dumbbells, which are more effective for working stabilization and balance in the shoulders. In addition to performing the bench press from the flat bench position, you can also perform on an incline. The incline dumbbell bench press is an excellent exercise for developing the upper chest and front shoulders.

1. Position yourself on a flat bench with the back flat and the feet on the floor.
2. Set your grip so that the hands are evenly spaced out from the middle of the bar. Use the bar's grip surface as a reference point. You may change the grip to emphasize different muscles. For instance, a wide grip works the outside of the chest while a close grip works the inside.
3. Using a spotter, raise the bar from the rack. When the weight is balanced above the chest, bend the elbows to move the bar toward the chest so that the weight is under control. Touch the middle of the chest with the bar and raise it back to the start position.
4. Make sure to breathe during the movement. Athletes typically breathe in on the descent of the bar and exhale on the upward movement.

SHOULDER PRESS

This exercise, along with the bench press, is one of the base strength movements for any athlete. The primary muscles worked are the deltoids, triceps, and trapezius. Athletes who perform overhead movements or who participate in sports requiring upper-body strength should perform this exercise. Volleyball, swimming, and basketball are some of the sports for which this exercise is especially beneficial. Perform the shoulder press using a straight barbell or dumbbell. We prefer dumbbells due to the increased stability and balance they require. You may perform this exercise seated or standing.

1. Start by holding two dumbbells at the front of the shoulders with the palms facing away from the body.
2. Slowly raise the dumbbells upward, keeping the weights balanced through the full range of movement.
3. Complete the upward movement by extending the arms so that the elbows are in full extension and the weight is overhead.
4. Return to the start position by performing a controlled downward movement of the weight.
5. Make sure to breathe throughout the movement and perform all repetitions through the fullest range of motion.

LAT PULL-DOWN

You typically perform this exercise on a machine to develop the latissimus dorsi, biceps, and brachioradialis muscles of the forearm. The "lats" are an important muscle group used for sports that require pulling, striking, and throwing movements such as softball, volleyball, and swimming. Athletes can change the emphasis of the muscles they work by changing their hand placement on the bar. A narrow underhand grip works the inside of the lats and the biceps while the wide overhand grip works the outside of the lats and forearms. We recommend pulling the bar to the front of the chest for close and wide grip movements. Pulling the weight behind the neck may place an added amount of stress on the neck.

1. Start by grasping the bar so that your grip is even.
2. Lean back slightly with the bar overhead and in front of you.
3. Pull the bar down to the upper portion of the chest and pause.
4. Finish the movement by slowly returning to the start position. Make sure to extend the arms at the top of the movement so that you fully activate the lats.

HANDSTAND PUSH-UP

Gymnasts and divers often use this exercise, but any athlete can use this exercise as a substitute for the shoulder press. It is excellent for developing total upper-body strength and balance and can help athletes with handstands and tumbling positions. The primary muscles it works include the deltoids, trapezius, and triceps. Perform this exercise against a wall or with a spotter.

1. Perform a handstand.
2. Start the movement by slowly bending the elbows to lower the body until the head taps the ground. Keep the body in a straight line by stabilizing the core muscles.
3. Complete the movement by pressing the body weight up until your elbows are fully extended.

POWER PUSH-UP

This exercise is excellent for developing explosive power in the upper body, including the chest and triceps muscles. Athletes with wrist or shoulder injuries should avoid the exercise due to its explosive nature.

1. Start the movement by lying flat on the ground on a thin mat, facedown, in the push-up position.
2. Perform a rapid push-up and press your body weight off the ground so that you are in the air with the arms fully extended. Keep the body in a straight line by stabilizing the muscles of the core.
3. As gravity returns your hands to the surface, control the body weight and bring the chest back to the floor.
4. Complete multiple repetitions is this manner. Be aggressive, but maintain a stable posture. If you are unable to keep good push-up form, do not perform this exercise until you obtain more upper-body strength and core stability.

SEATED ROW

This exercise is great for any athlete to develop the middle back musculature, particularly the rhomboids and scapular stabilizers, as well as the biceps. This exercise is typically performed on a machine but may also be performed with a partner, with each of you holding the end of a thick bungee cord or towel. Not only is it a great strength exercise, but it is one of the multijoint movements that links many of the upper body's muscles together to develop posture and stability (we call this kinetic linking).

1. Start by sitting up with tall posture. You will typically be seated in front of a column pulley system.
2. With the hands holding a bar or rowing handle, slowly pull the designated weight toward you, so that the bar touches your lower chest. Keep your back flat and knees bent.
3. Complete the movement by returning the weight to the start position in a controlled fashion.

BUNGEE SWING FOR GOLF

This exercise is designed to help golfers develop strength, stability, and endurance at the core, but other athletes may find it useful as well, especially softball pitchers and field hockey players. You may also perform this exercise on balance discs for added balance and stability.

1. Attach a bungee cord to an immovable object or surface and stand six to eight feet away.
2. Start in the "address position" (golfer's starting stance). Find a comfortable stance where the feet are hip-width apart, the chest is over the feet, the back is flat, and the arms are holding the bungee cord like a club.
3. Step away from the bungee so that there is enough tension to provide adequate resistance. While in the address position and holding the bungee at the midline of the body, slowly move the hands back and away from the midline until your arms make a hinge.
4. Complete a forward arcing half swing, keeping the front arm straight as it passes the midline. Make sure to keep the core stable throughout the movement while tightening the obliques.
5. Return to the start position and repeat the designated number of repetitions.

PHYSIOBALL SWIMMER

This exercise develops strength and stability in the back extensor muscles and gluteals. It is also great to start workouts with this exercise as a warm-up. Athletes with postural problems should include this exercise in their daily regimen. Use a 55- to 65-centimeter diameter physioball that has a burst-resistant rating for safety purposes.

1. Position the body facedown on the ball with the ball at the center point of the body. This is your balance point.
2. Extend the legs out and arms overhead. You will need to place the left hand and the right foot on the ground for balance. With the left hand and right foot on the ground, raise the right hand and left foot upward while keeping the body stable.
3. Perform this alternating movement for the designated amount of repetitions. If you cannot maintain balance try a smaller ball.

RICE: THREE WAY

This exercise is excellent for developing hand, wrist, and forearm strength and endurance. You will need two five-gallon buckets placed side-by-side and filled with brown rice. Fill the buckets two-thirds to three-quarters full. You may also use beans or marbles for different resistance, but rice seems to work best. Perform this exercise at the end of your workout.

1. Start by placing the hands in each bucket so that one-inch past the wrist is submerged in the rice.
2. For the first set squeeze the rice by simply opening and closing the hand. Make sure to keep the hand submerged for the whole set.
3. For the second set, squeeze the rice and twist the hands to the right as if closing a jar.
4. For the third set, squeeze the rice and twist the hands to the left as if opening a jar.
5. Perform one set of each direction for 25 to 50 repetitions each set.

If you are looking for a routine specifically designed to build strength in the shoulder and to prevent injury (or to rehabilitate from an existing shoulder injury), chapter 9 provides a solid, focused upper-extremity workout for those purposes. Use it on its own or in coordination with your strength, power, and conditioning routine.

Hip, Knee, and Ankle Stabilization

The initial goal for any athlete is health and longevity throughout her career. Lower-extremity health (of the knees in particular) is especially important because female athletes are at greater risk than male athletes for knee injuries. Fortunately, specific training can help females strengthen and stabilize the hips, knees, and ankles. This chapter discusses the anatomy of the lower extremity and the specific factors that predispose women to greater risk for serious injury, particularly of the knee. Finally, we present specific exercises designed to promote strength and stability in the lower extremity.

Recent research shows significant differences between the rates of injury in female versus male athletes, both for those participating in the same sports and for female athletes across the board. Several factors attempt to explain this phenomenon, including the anatomical and physiological differences between the sexes and the recent explosion in the number of competitive female athletes and their increased level of play. Both of these contribute to the number of injuries.

- It is estimated that 30,000 high school and college-aged females will sustain knee injuries in 2004.
- Female athletes injure their knees at a rate three to five times higher than men.
- Female basketball and soccer players sustain three to four times more knee injuries than men who participate in the same sports.
- In the 1990s, 1.4 million women tore their anterior cruciate ligaments (ACLs), two times the rate of the same injury in the 1980s.
- Data presented by the NCAA shows that women volleyball players injured their ACLs 73 percent more often in game situations than in practice.
- Most injuries occur during deceleration, when an athlete is stopping, cutting, or landing.

From this evidence we see an alarming trend that continues to increase as the level of play and the intensity of women in athletics also increase. The fact that so many female athletes are injured during the high-intensity environment of games or competition suggests that their bodies are not ready to meet these demands. Physical preparation goes beyond general conditioning. The primary issue is muscle strength, stability, and proprioception (balance). To understand how to correct this problem we must first understand why women athletes are more susceptible to lower-extremity injuries, specifically knee injuries.

Current research shows that women tend to have smaller ACLs than men do, which increases their risk for injury. Because a woman's ACL is smaller, and she tends to have less overall muscular strength to support the knee than her male counterparts do, a woman's ACL is at a greater risk of tearing because of the load placed on it during sport. Moreover, men and women have different quadriceps angles (Q-angles). The Q-angle is the angle of the femur as it enters the hip socket. Women's Q-angles are wider than men's. Although no concrete evidence indicates that the Q-angle plays a major role in ACL tears, evidence shows that it contributes to patellofemoral tracking problems and anterior knee pain. Perhaps more important, the patellar notch on the female athlete is smaller than on men, and evidence shows that the ACL can get caught and sliced in the notch. And the wider Q-angle makes the ACL more vulnerable to tearing in the notch.

A biomechanical problem women face that contributes to knee injuries is an imbalance between the quadriceps and hamstring muscle groups. Women tend to rely more heavily on their quadriceps muscle group for primary knee strength and stability rather than create a balance between the quadriceps and hamstrings. Women also tend to land more flat-footed and with straighter legs than men do. This practice increases the ground force and contributes to increased force on the joints—not just on the knees, but on the ankles and hips also.

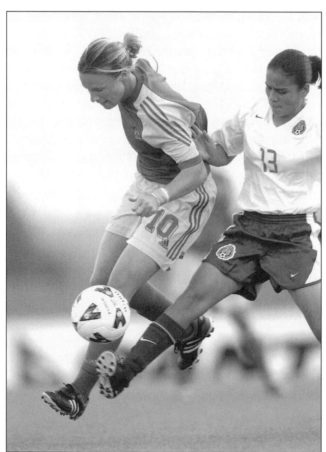

Balanced, well-trained muscles of the lower extremity help keep knees healthy.

Evidence shows that female athletes need to enhance their neuromuscular control to prevent ankle, knee, and hip injuries. Studies show that athletes who had increased their performance in drills that tested balance and neuromuscular control were less likely to become injured.

Another factor that likely contributes to women's more frequent lower-body injuries is that girls tend not to receive athletic training that focuses on the basics early enough in their athletic careers. Coaches need to prepare young athletes for the demands of athletics with basics such as form running, fast-feet drills, stopping, starting, jumping, and strength training. Boys tend to receive this type of training earlier through organized sports than girls do. For example, in sports like gymnastics for both girls and boys, because there is a lot of physical and technical training, we can surmise that the higher rate of injuries is most likely due to the demands of the sport and to anatomical differences. In sports like soccer and basketball, however, where there is a very high number of participants, we see increases in injury rates for female athletes more due to deficiencies in physical and technical preparation. (We also tend to see a greater number of male high school athletes in the weight room at an earlier time in their careers.) We know that because of girls' anatomical and biomechanical differences, they need this training. Many child development experts suggest that a child's greatest opportunity for motor learning occurs between the ages of 8 and 12. Once we miss this opportunity to train the basics, it becomes more difficult to "unteach" the bad habits and correct the neuromuscular deficiencies.

The exercises in this chapter give you the tools to strengthen the lower extremity to help overcome some of these deficiencies and also to increase the length of your sport career. But first, a basic understanding of this part of the body and its function during sport movements will help you better understand your lower extremity and its training needs.

STRUCTURE OF THE LOWER EXTREMITY

Bones are responsible for structure, stability, attachment surface, and lever systems by which all movement occurs. Bones also protect vital internal organs. Ligaments attach bone to bone and act as the primary stabilizers of the bones in the hip, knee, and ankle joints. When ligaments (such as the ACL in the knee) are torn, the stability of the joint is compromised. Ligaments do not have a rich blood supply, so when they tear, healing is slow. Often surgery is required. Unlike muscles, ligaments cannot be strengthened through training. This is why strengthening the surrounding muscles is crucial. Increased strength in muscles provides another source of stabilization for the knee so that less strain is placed on the ligaments.

Tendons attach muscle to bone. Their insertion into the bone allows the muscles to move the bone. Tendons have a greater blood supply than ligaments and cartilage and therefore usually heal more quickly. Overuse syndrome often occurs in tendons because of their position of attachment and the dynamic load placed on them.

Cartilage provides surface area for bone interface and acts as a shock absorber in the joint. Like ligaments, the blood supply to cartilage is poor, creating an environment for slow healing. Maintaining the integrity of cartilage is vital for an athlete's longevity. The phrase *bone on bone* refers to the breakdown in knee cartilage that predisposes the knee to all kinds of other problems. Cartilage comes in two separate forms, each has a different function.

Hyaline cartilage is found on the surface of long bone endings and on some flat bones like the patella. It works as a lubricant so that the movement of the joint is more fluid. It also protects the joint surfaces. When this cartilage is worn down over time, athletes can develop pain, crepitus (grinding), and even bone spurs. Muscular imbalance caused by lack of strength in the supporting muscles contributes to wearing of the hyaline cartilage. An example of this cartilage is found on the underside of the patella bone where it meets with the femoral heads.

Fibrocartilage is a strong fibrous soft tissue called meniscus. The menisci are found in the knee and serve two purposes. Unlike slippery hyaline cartilage that works as a lubricant, the menisci absorb shock during landing, jumping, running, or changes of direction—any movement that loads the knee joint. Their second function is to provide surface area for the connection between the femur and tibia so that there is a good fit at the joint. The medial and lateral menisci are often torn with twisting or extreme compressive forces. These injuries are hard to prevent because of their traumatic nature, but maintaining strong musculature may provide protection during situations that produce extreme compression and torsion at the knee joint.

The hip is a ball-and-socket joint composed of hyaline cartilage. It is the strongest and most durable joint in the body. Deficiencies in strength that weaken this joint can affect the athlete's core strength and affect other joints in the kinetic chain—especially the knee and ankle. Many competitive athletes experience deficiencies in their flexibility or strength of the muscles around this joint; these deficiencies show up as imbalances in the pelvic girdle and can even be responsible for low back problems.

We discuss the musculature of the hip in more detail in chapter 5 because the hip joint plays an important role in stabilizing the core of the body during many movements. It is extremely important for female athletes to focus on the gluteal, hamstring, and inner quadriceps muscles to keep the hip joint healthy. These muscles help maintain proper balance between the strong opposing muscles of the lower extremity (see table 4.1).

Table 4.1 Muscles of the Hip, Knee, and Ankle and Their Functions

Group	Muscle	Primary function
Hip and knee	Iliopsoas (includes the iliacus, psoas minor, and psoas major)	Flexion and rotation of the spine Flexion, adduction, and external rotation of the hip
	Psoas minor	Flexion of the pelvis
	Iliacus Sartorius Tensor fasciae latae Pectineus Piriformis Quadratus femoris	Flexion, adduction, and external rotation of the femur
	Gluteus medius	Abduction, flexion, and internal rotation of the femur
	Gluteus minimus	Abduction, flexion, extension, and internal rotation of the femur
	Semitendinosus Semimembranosus Gluteus maximus	Extension, adduction, and internal rotation of the femur
	Rectus femoris Vastus lateralis Gracilis Vastus medialis	Knee extension, hip flexion
Ankle	Gastrocnemius Soleus	Plantar flexion of the foot
	Sartorius	Dorsiflexion of the foot
	Peroneals	Eversion and dorsiflexion of the foot

Many of the muscles discussed earlier also affect the actions of the knee. The muscles of the knee joint perform four major actions. They act as flexors, extensors, rotators, and gliders. The quadriceps group (vastus lateralis, vastus medialis, vastus intermedius, and rectus femoris) are the primary extensors of the knee. The hamstring group (semitendinosus, semimembranosus, and biceps femoris), the sartorius, and the gracilis muscles act as flexors of the knee. The sartorius and gracilis muscles aid in the rotation of the knee. The muscles surrounding the knee are responsible for moving the bones around the joint, and they also act as secondary stabilizers to the ligaments. The muscles that are primary to the hip include the gluteus maximus, medius, and minimus; piriformis; quadratus; illiacus; and sartorius. These muscles control flexion, extension, and external and internal rotation of the leg on the hip. Illustrated in figures 4.1*a* through *c* are the major structures of the hip and knee.

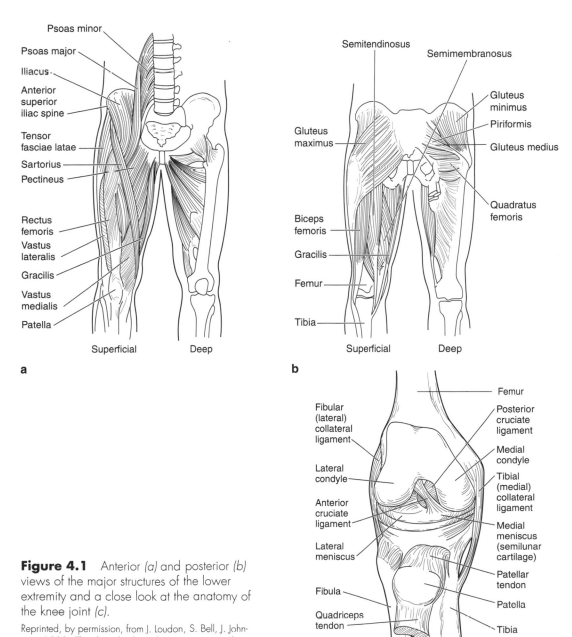

Figure 4.1 Anterior *(a)* and posterior *(b)* views of the major structures of the lower extremity and a close look at the anatomy of the knee joint *(c)*.

Reprinted, by permission, from J. Loudon, S. Bell, J. Johnston, 1998, *The clinical orthopedic assessment guide* (Champaign, IL: Human Kinetics), 155, 161.

The joints of the ankle help connect the tarsal bones of the foot. Although we won't delve into the ankle joint in great detail here, note that many of the standing exercises that develop hip and knee stability also strengthen the muscles supporting the ankle. While the lower extremity gets its power from the knee and hip joints, the ankle's important role is in stabilizing and balancing the lower extremity. The foot and ankle are the intricate starting point for the kinetic chain of lower-extremity movements; thus any deficiency in foot and ankle strength can result in knee and hip injuries.

EXERCISES FOR A STRONG AND HEALTHY LOWER EXTREMITY

The remainder of this chapter provides specific training exercises designed to increase the strength and stability of your hips, knees, and ankles. In later chapters we present jump programs, power programs, and other specific programs that further strengthen the lower extremity and that are designed to make you a better athlete in your particular sport. The exercises that follow can be used as base strengthening work (both in-season and off-season) for any sport. See chapter 9 for ways to incorporate these important lower-extremity exercises into your specific sport program.

As you work on the exercises that follow, keep in mind several primary goals for any lower-extremity program designed for female athletes.

- Increase the strength and stability of the joint
- Increase the athletic capabilities of the athlete by including multijoint exercises that incorporate functional movements
- Develop hamstring strength
- Incorporate exercises requiring balance

BASIC STRENGTH EXERCISES

When beginning a new exercise focus first on technique; do not be concerned with the amount of weight you are lifting. When doing free weight lifts, start by lifting just the Olympic bar, perfect your form, and *then* add weight. If you can't maintain good technique, reduce the amount of weight until you can. Then gradually increase the weight, maintaining proper technique.

BACK SQUAT

The squat focuses on the deficiencies of the lower extremity that we discussed at the beginning of this chapter and is an important multijoint exercise that provides the functional muscle development women need for sport. Multijoint exercises are those in which two or more joints are involved in the movement, and they usually involve large muscle groups. Most multijoint exercises are functional; that is, they simulate the movements that athletes do, incorporating an element of balance and center-of-gravity work. For example, this squat exercise uses muscles that cross the hip, knee, and ankle joints. The knee extension on a machine, however, is a single-joint exercise; it involves muscles of the knee joint only. The squat helps develop a great base for the serious athlete in any sport looking to take her training to the next level.

1. Place the bar on the upper back (trapezius). Set the handgrip so that each hand is an even distance from the neck.
2. Position the feet just outside the hips with the toes pointed out slightly. Maintain a flat-footed stance throughout the movement.
3. Keep the head up slightly and the back flat throughout the movement as you bend the knees, squatting until the upper legs are parallel to the floor.
4. Use a weight that allows you to squat until the upper legs are parallel to the floor using proper technique. Keep in mind that depth is more important than weight when developing strength.
5. Work to develop flexibility in the calf–Achilles region.

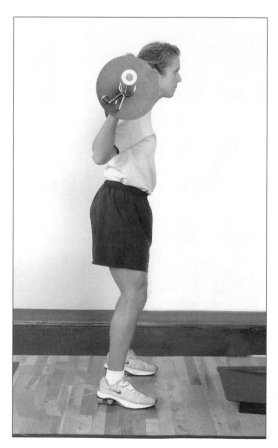 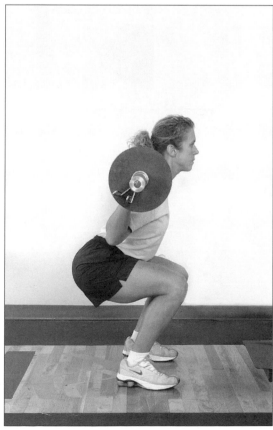

FRONT SQUAT

The front squat works the quadriceps, gluteals, hamstrings, and lumbar muscles. It is an excellent exercise for developing the front of the thigh and is essential for progressing to the Olympic lifts (see chapter 7).

1. Place the bar on the front shoulders (anterior deltoids).
2. Find a comfortable hand position. Grasp the bar with the palms facing up and the elbows high. Many athletes need to work on stretching their shoulders and wrists in order to develop the proper technique
3. Position the feet just outside the hips with the toes pointed out slightly.
4. Keep the head up slightly and the back arched slightly throughout the movement as you bend the knees to squat until the thighs are parallel to the floor.
5. Use a weight that allows you to squat until the upper legs are parallel to the floor using proper technique. Again, keep in mind that the depth of the squat is more important than the weight.

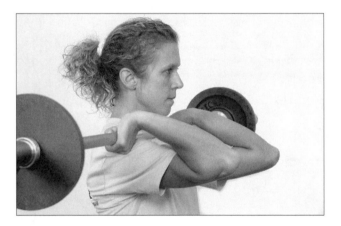

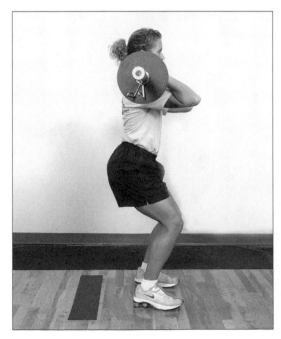
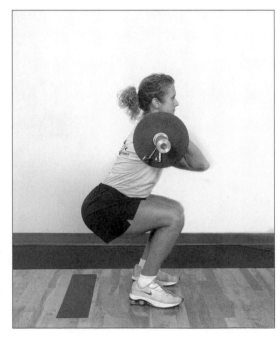

ROMANIAN DEADLIFT

The Romanian deadlift, commonly referred to as a RDL, is an excellent exercise for building strength and stability in the muscles of the back as well as the hamstrings and the gluteals. It is also a great exercise to master before moving on to Olympic-style weightlifting, which includes lifts such as the hang clean and power clean (see pages 127 and 129 in chapter 7).

1. The movement begins with the feet in a neutral position about hip-width apart. Distribute the weight evenly on the feet throughout the motion. Keep the knees slightly bent, not locked. This bending will result in slight hip flexion. Keep the back slightly arched. Pulling the shoulders back and keeping the head in a forward, neutral position will help hold this position throughout the movement.

2. In this position, hold a barbell close to the body with a grip of about shoulder width. Initiate the movement as if the body were broken into two parts: the upper and lower.

3. Slowly drop the upper half as if there were a hinge at the hips. There is no additional flexion at the knees or ankles. The barbell should maintain a close path of motion with the body and be lowered only until you feel a moderate stretch in either the hamstrings or the low back.

4. At this point, the motion should change direction. Maintaining a flat back and flexed knees, retrace the path of the barbell to the start position.

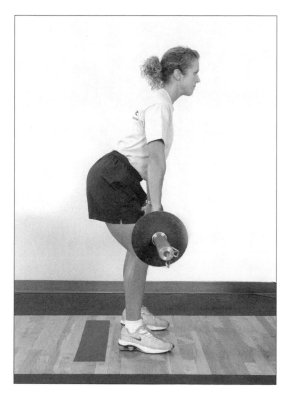
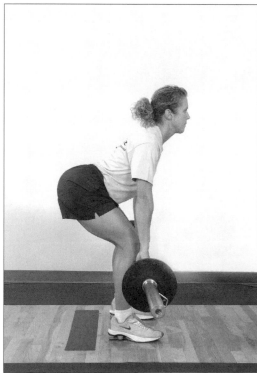

TRADITIONAL DEADLIFT

The deadlift is an exercise used by itself and as a training step in learning the power clean (see page 129). Executing this exercise properly teaches an athlete how to pick the bar up from the floor safely and control it. The exercise emphasizes the muscles of the back and the legs.

1. Place the feet about hip-width apart.
2. Stabilize the muscles of the core, pull back the shoulders, and keep the head in a neutral position as you lower the body as if sitting in a chair. If at any time during this movement the low back starts to round or the shoulders start to fall forward, work on more flexibility in the hamstrings and the erector muscles of the back before proceeding with this exercise. While you are developing flexibility, be sure to use lighter weights and to perform the exercise in front of a mirror to be sure you are performing it correctly.
3. With the arms relaxed and elbows rotated out to the sides, grip the bar.
4. Place your weight on the back one-third of the feet, keeping the entire foot in contact with the floor throughout the movement.
5. Lifting the bar begins with extension at the hip. The knees and ankles will follow. Keep the chest forward with the shoulders pulled back.
6. Lift the bar until the body is in a straight, upright position.
7. Reverse the movement to return the bar to the ground. Keeping a rigid back and focusing on the hips is essential throughout this movement.

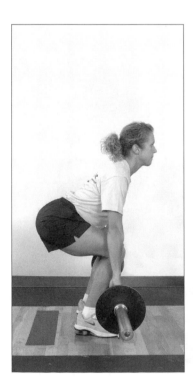 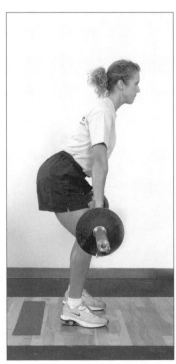 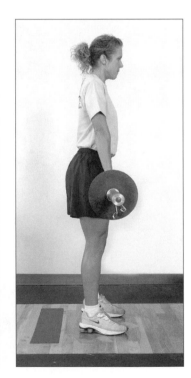

LEG PRESS WITH ADDUCTION

The leg press works the quadriceps and the adductors (inner thigh muscles). You can perform the leg press using machines or sleds. Squeezing a ball between the legs during the movement activates the adductors and vastus medialis during knee extension. The isometric contraction of the adductors stabilizes the hips throughout the range of motion (ROM).

1. Place a small medicine ball (3 to 5 pounds or 1.5 to 2 kilograms) between the inner thighs.
2. Keep the low back in contact with the back pad of the machine.
3. Grasp the handles.
4. Press the weight forward while squeezing the ball until full contraction. Straighten the legs, but do not completely lock the knees.
5. Return to the start position slowly with the knees flexed at 90 degrees.

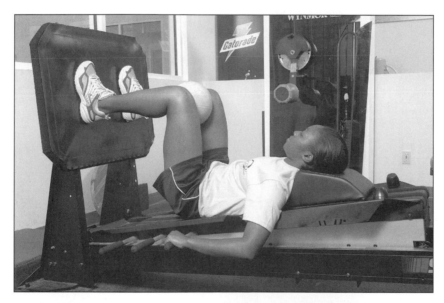

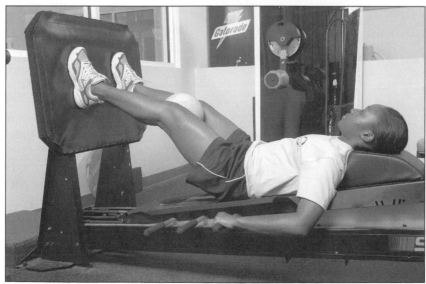

SINGLE-LEG KNEE EXTENSION

The knee extension is a single-joint exercise that develops the inner quadriceps muscle group. While this is not a functional, multijoint exercise, strengthening this muscle group is important because it will provide stability during the initial knee extension and flexion during deceleration, cutting, and jumping. Strong muscles act as secondary stabilizers.

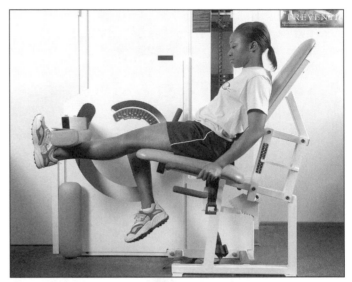

1. Sit at the machine, and position the knee so that it is lined up with the axis of rotation of the movement arm.
2. Extend the leg so that the inner thigh is contracted fully. Hold for 1 to 2 seconds.
3. Slowly return to the start position.

SINGLE-LEG HAMSTRING CURL

The hamstring curl is another single-joint exercise that is especially beneficial for female athletes. Isolating the hamstring (which is what this exercise focuses on) provides a base of strength for the knee and helps build a secondary support system for the ACL.

1. Lie on the machine, and position the knee so that it is lined up with the axis of rotation of the movement arm.
2. Keep the hips flat against the surface of the machine.
3. Flex the leg at the knee so that the hamstrings are contracted fully. Hold for 1 to 2 seconds.
4. Slowly return to the start position.

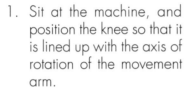

GLUTE–HAM: STRAIGHT LEG

The glute–ham: straight leg (also called the back extension), performed in a straight-leg position, is one of the best ways to isolate the upper hamstrings. It also works the gluteals and the lumbar muscle (erector spinae) group. Two primary muscle groups of the hip and knee joints that promote healthy knees in female athletes are the gluteals and hamstrings. The gluteals provide power and stability for explosive cuts and turns and are linked to the knee by the hamstring muscle group, which provides power for sprinting and stability for stopping. This exercise should be a mainstay in your strength training program.

1. Position the body facedown on the bench so that the prominent bone on the hip is just to the front of the pad. A bench with a rounded pad is the best option. A proper fit allows the feet to press flat on the platform.
2. Cross the arms over the chest or place them behind the head.
3. With the legs anchored, knees straight, and body position parallel to the floor, slowly lower the upper body so that it is almost perpendicular to the floor.
4. Return to the start position where the body is parallel to the floor, keeping the upper body rigid throughout the motion.
5. As your strength increases, grasp a weight or medicine ball to the chest while you complete the movement.
6. You can modify this exercise to include the obliques by adding a twist at the top of the motion.

This exercise can also be done with the knees bent, thighs flat to the pad (must be done on a half-moon glute–ham bench pad), and body parallel to the floor. In this case you raise the body up into a perpendicular position and return to start. This takes the hamstrings out and isolates the lumbar and gluteal musculature (see chapter 5, page 87).

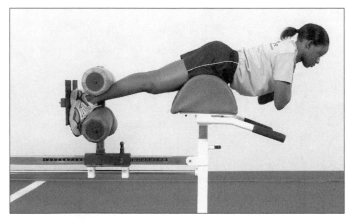

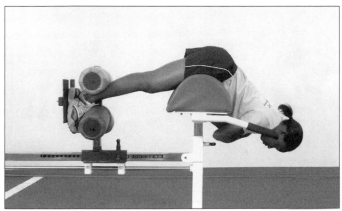

FUNCTIONAL STRENGTH EXERCISES

Functional strength training is the bridge between low-intensity (basic strength) and high-intensity (explosive strength and power) work. Many athletes train for power prematurely, which puts them at greater risk for injury because they have not built a proper base or performed functional work. The base exercises listed in the basic-strength section lay the foundation for the greater demands of functional work. The exercises that follow are multijoint and functional.

Sometimes extreme movements during competition place female athletes in precarious positions that can result in injury. These functional exercises work not only on strength, but also focus on improving the balance and body position awareness that can help prevent injury. They also mimic many of the movement patterns performed in competition. Functional exercises stimulate the same muscles that produce athletic movements. A primary benefit is that they stimulate the nerves that affect muscle firing and provide the muscle memory needed to perform difficult tasks. Although it provides benefits, a single-joint exercise like the knee extension may not prepare the nervous system in the same way that a multijoint exercise like a walking lunge, power lunge, or weight transfer exercise does.

WALKING LUNGE

The walking lunge strengthens the hamstrings, gluteals, and quadriceps muscles and can be performed without weights or with a barbell, dumbbells, or other weight implements like medicine balls or weighted inner tubes.

1. Place the weight directly over the shoulders.
2. Start with the head up and the back straight. Maintain this position throughout the movement.
3. Step forward far enough that the knee is over the ball of the foot at the end of the movement.
4. Repeat the movement by shifting the weight to the opposite leg and stepping forward with that leg.
5. Perform this movement at a controlled pace through the fullest range of motion possible.

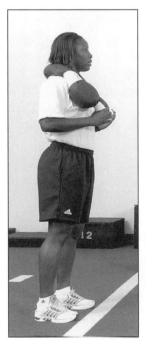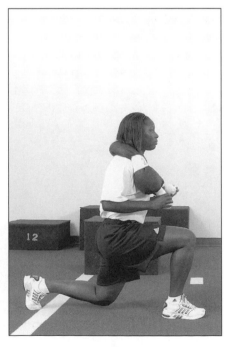

You can increase the intensity of the walking lunge by performing power lunges. The power lunge is performed in the same way as the walking lunge with the addition of an explosive skip step upon the elevation of the forward knee. At step 4 described earlier, come out of the lunge (head up, knee over midfoot, upper body perpendicular) by stepping with the opposite foot. During the step, drive the knee upward so that the momentum elevates the body off the ground. Land on the takeoff leg and go into the next lunge. This creates a lunge with a power skip.

FORWARD BOX STEP-UP

Box step-ups are excellent exercises for developing functional strength in the lower extremity, primarily the hamstrings, gluteals, and quadriceps. Set the box height so that the upper thigh is parallel to the ground when the foot is on the box. This will ensure a full range of motion and safety for the knee.

1. Place a barbell or weighted bag across the back of the shoulders (or hold a dumbbell at each side).
2. Stand facing the box.
3. Raise the right leg onto the box so that the foot rests completely on the box.
4. Press your weight up using the right leg only. Do not jump or use momentum.
5. Finish the upward movement by standing on the box in a straight body position.
6. Complete the exercise by lowering the left leg first, followed by the right.
7. Repeat and switch legs.

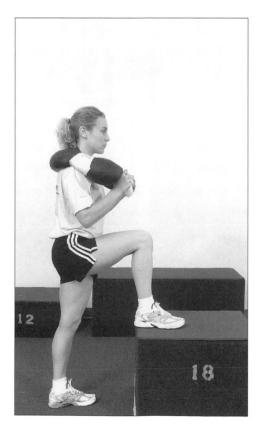
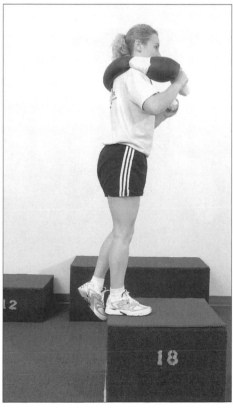

SIDE BOX STEP-UP

This exercise works the hamstrings, gluteals, and quadriceps muscles as well as the adductors (inner thigh). The adductors are extremely important in stabilizing the hips during cutting and while changing direction. They provide a powerful leg swing during kicking movements and flex, rotate, and extend the thigh.

1. Place a barbell or weighted bag across the back of the shoulders (or hold a dumbbell at each side).
2. Stand with the left side of the body next to the box.
3. Raise the left leg up so that the foot rests completely on the box. Be sure the left foot turns outward slightly to protect the knee.
4. Press your weight up using the left leg only. Do not jump or use momentum.
5. Finish the upward movement by standing on the box in a straight body position.
6. Complete the exercise by lowering the right leg first followed by the left.
7. Repeat and switch legs.

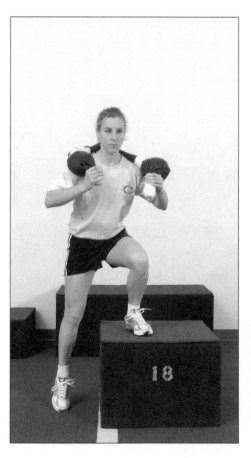
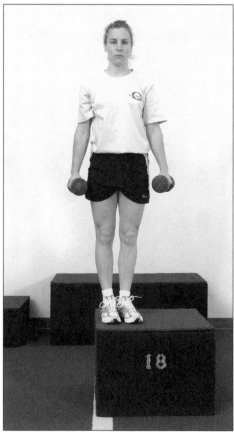

SIDE LUNGE

Side lunges develop the hamstrings, gluteals, and adductor muscles, which are involved in diagonal movements. This exercise improves the ability to decelerate.

1. Place a weighted bag or barbell on the upper back.
2. Stand with the head forward and back flat. Step right at a 30- to 45-degree angle until the upper thigh of the lead leg is parallel to the ground.
3. Land so that the knee is over the ball of the foot in the finish position.
4. Do not let the knee move past the foot.
5. Keep the back leg slightly bent. Keep the upper body perpendicular to the ground.
6. Finish the movement by pressing back up to the standing position.
7. Alternate legs with each lunge or switch legs after finishing a complete set on one leg.

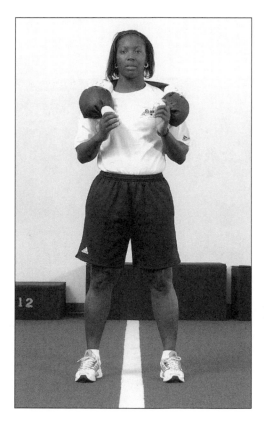 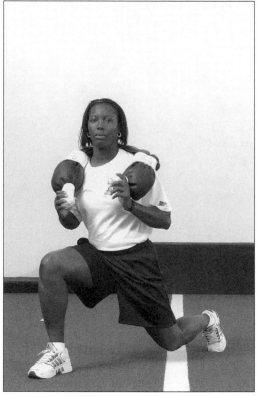

THREE-WAY WEIGHT TRANSFER

Weight transfers are a variation of the lunge but focus primarily on balance and muscular control as the movement is completed. They work all the lower-extremity muscles as well as the lumbar and abdominal muscles. This is another exercise that strengthens the legs to help stabilize the body during the deceleration phase of any movement. It prepares female athletes for the movements that can cause injury. Weight transfers can be performed forward, on a diagonal of 30 to 60 degrees, or directly to the side.

1. Start in a standing position. You can use just your body weight or light dumbbells.
2. With the hands straight out at shoulder height (with or without dumbbells), take a short hop step onto the left leg.
3. Land on the left foot in a half-lunge position with the back foot straight and off the ground (similar to the scale position in gymnastics). Maintain your balance holding this position for 1 to 2 seconds.
4. Complete the exercise by hopping backward to the standing start position.
5. Complete all repetitions on the same leg, and then perform the exercise on the other leg.

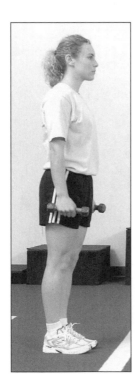 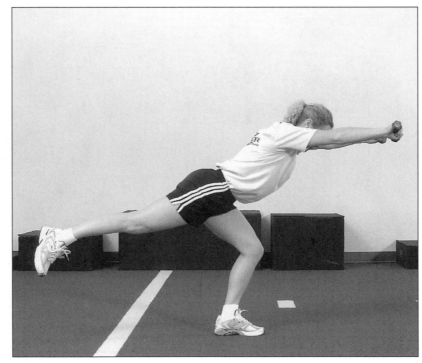

STANDING TWO-WAY CALF RAISE

The calf muscles are composed of the gastrocnemius and the soleus. The gastrocnemius is part of the knee complex of muscles. It attaches above the knee and actually crosses the joint, playing a role in knee flexion. The standing two-way calf raise works primarily the gastrocnemius muscle in the back of the lower leg. If you wish to work the soleus muscle, performing this exercise in a seated position.

1. Start in a standing position on a two-inch platform with the toes turned outward slightly. You can hold dumbbells, a barbell, or a wall, or you can use a calf machine.
2. Slowly elevate the heels as high as they will go until the calves are fully contracted.
3. Hold at the top of the movement for 1 to 2 seconds, and slowly return to the starting position.
4. Complete the second set with the toes pointed inward slightly.

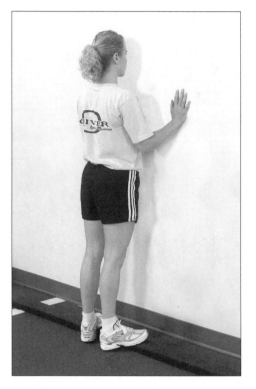

SHUFFLE SQUAT

In addition to the side lunge and side box step-up, which work on inner and outer thigh muscles, the shuffle squat is another great exercise that incorporates the adductor and abductor muscles of the thighs as well as the gluteal muscles, quadriceps, and hamstrings.

1. Start in a standing position with the feet shoulder-width apart.
2. Perform a squat movement, keeping the back straight and bending at the knees.
3. From the squat position, take a power step to the right as you move upward and outward from the squat.
4. Reset the feet in the squat position.
5. Perform the movement for 15 to 20 reps for each leg.

All of the exercises detailed in this chapter can be found in the sport-specific programs provided in chapter 9. By placing the appropriate exercises within the programs for specific sports, you can customize your program to work those lower-extremity muscles that will be most beneficial for your sports performance.

Core and Balance Development

The core is more than just the physical center of the body. Its strength actually dictates athleticism. The core is an intricate system of musculature of the trunk—including the abdominal and back muscles—and the hips. An athlete with a solid, strong core displays balance, agility, proprioceptive awareness, strength, power, and endurance—all are imperative to raising any sport-specific skill to a high level of athleticism. For example, a softball player uses a well-trained core to transfer power from the legs to the upper body to swing the bat. A volleyball player uses it to make a kill. A sprinter transfers power from the arms to the legs through the core, and a swimmer uses it to make a smooth turn at the end of the lane.

Just about every sport relies on a strong and stable core. Yet attention to the core area is often overlooked or trained with less intensity than it should be. Usually the primary reason for an undertrained core is that the core-strength training was incorporated into the wrong phase of the training program. Core strengthening should be included in a training program in the same way that weight training and conditioning are: based on periodized training and set up so that an athlete can meet her core-strengthening goals.

STRUCTURE OF THE CORE

As discussed in chapters 3 and 4, bones provide the structure and foundation for the attachment of soft tissue such as muscles and tendons that move bony structures through varying ranges of movement. The bones of the core are composed of two general regions—the upper and lower core.

The bones of the trunk or upper core region are the spine and its vertebrae. The primary muscle of the trunk involving flexion of the spine is the rectus abdominis. The internal and external obliques allow for flexion of the spine but are best known as rotators of the trunk. The quadratus lumborum is one of the primary muscles that link the spine and hips. It is responsible for extension and lateral flexion of the spine and may be an area of weakness for many athletes who do not develop their core

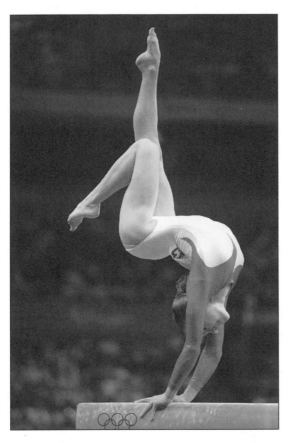

This Olympic gymnast demonstrates the core stability, balance, strength, and endurance it takes to excel in her sport.

musculature. It is important to work the flexors and extensors equally to maintain muscular balance.

The hips make up the lower half of the core and include the bony structures of the illium, ischium, pubis, and femur bones. The areas of muscle and tendon attachment on these structures are crucial in determining movement around the hips. The gluteus maximus and gluteus medius muscles are primarily responsible for abduction, flexion, extension, and internal rotation of the femur on the hip joint. The sartorius, quadratus femoris, and piriformis link the femur to the core, allowing flexion, adduction, and external rotation of the femur on the hip. The illiopsoas is one of the crucial muscles that link the hip and the spine. It allows for flexion and rotation of the spine and flexion, adduction, and external rotation of the hip.

Table 5.1 details the functions of the various muscles of the trunk and hip. Figure 5.1 *a* and *b* on page 82 shows the muscles of the core. Refer to figures 4.1 *a* and *b* (page 63) for an anatomical drawing showing the muscles of the hip.

In addition to the functions listed in table 5.1, core muscles also help stabilize the body. Most sport movements are synergistic—a pair or group of muscles work together to perform the movement. While one muscle or a group of muscles is contracting, others must stabilize. For example, when a batter prepares and swings at a ball, muscles contract throughout the body. While the legs transfer power from the lower body to the upper body, the muscles of the trunk contract and stabilize the body throughout the movement. The stabilizers are necessary for complex, explosive, or precise movements. A rigid torso is necessary for this transfer of power in many sport movements such as throwing, jumping, hurdling, swimming, and tumbling. Examine almost any movement in sport and you will notice how important the core's role is in the movement or in stabilizing the body for the movement. Many movements that we take for granted such as walking, getting up from a chair, and getting into a car rely on the trunk stabilizers.

The muscles involved in any movement are considered prime movers (agonists), opposing muscles (antagonists), and assisting muscles (synergists). The agonist muscle is the primary force behind the dynamic movement. The antagonists and synergists are responsible for stabilizing the joint during explosive and precise sport movements.

The hips are the most important core stabilizer; many of the most powerful movements in sport are initiated with hip extension, which uses the gluteus maximus as the prime mover, the psoas and rectus femoris as the antagonists, and the erector spinae and biceps femoris as the synergists.

Table 5.1 Muscles of the Core and Their Functions

Group	Muscle	Primary function
Trunk	Rectus abdominis	Flexion of the spine and pelvic girdle flexion
	Internal obliques Transversus abdominis	Flexion and rotation of the spine
	External obliques	Flexion and rotation of the spine and pelvic girdle flexion
	Iliocostalis lumborum Multifidus	Extension and rotation of the spine
	Sacrospinalis	Extension, lateral flexion, and rotation of the spine
	Quadratus lumborum	Extension and lateral flexion of the spine
Hip	Iliopsoas	Flexion and rotation of the spine Flexion, adduction, and external rotation of the hip
	Psoas minor	Flexion of pelvis
	Iliacus Sartorius Tensor fasciae latae Pectineus Piriformis Quadratus femoris	Flexion, adduction, and external rotation of the femur
	Gluteus medius	Abduction, flexion, and internal rotation of the femur
	Gluteus minimus	Abduction, flexion, extension, and internal rotation of the femur
	Semitendinosus Semimembranosus Gluteus maximus	Extension, adduction, and internal rotation of the femur

In hip extension, if the erector spinae, biceps femoris, psoas, and rectus femoris are not trained to stabilize the movement, repetitive hip extensions may result in poor performance of the gluteus maximus and lead to pain or an overuse injury. The same is true for hip flexion, hip abduction, and hip adduction. Repeated movements develop neural patterns. When you kick a ball repeatedly, you don't have to think about how to kick the ball before initiating the action. But if you have been kicking with incorrect technique for a while, you will have a difficult time correcting this movement because the muscles and nerves have developed a pattern for kicking that way. Improper stabilization over time can develop improper neural patterns, making them difficult to correct. Stretching and learning to fire stabilizing muscle groups can take months of specific training. When correcting technique, it is important to progress slowly. Just as you learned to kick correctly over time, it takes time to revise technical movements, even stabilizing actions. Executing a movement correctly from the beginning is more efficient and effective in the long run and may decrease the potential for acute and chronic injury.

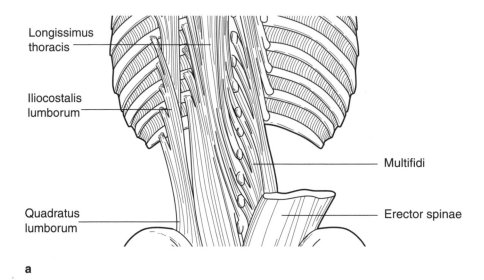

- Longissimus thoracis
- Iliocostalis lumborum
- Quadratus lumborum
- Multifidi
- Erector spinae

a

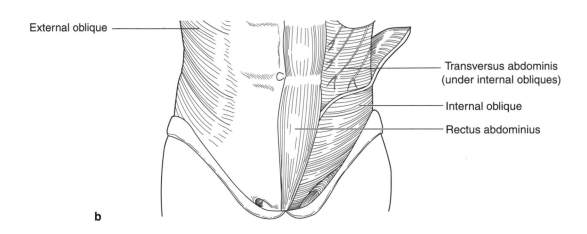

- External oblique
- Transversus abdominis (under internal obliques)
- Internal oblique
- Rectus abdominius

b

Figure 5.1 Muscles of the core.

Reprinted, by permission, from J. Loudon, S. Bell, J. Johnston, 1998, *The clinical orthopedic assessment guide* (Champaign, IL: Human Kinetics), 62.

Strength and flexibility are partners in sport. Sport movements require the joint and muscle to contract and stabilize through an active range of motion beyond what is considered normal. This level of flexibility is different than passive flexibility, or how much a muscle can be stretched while relaxed. During sport movements, the muscles and joint capsules must be supple while contracting and especially while stabilizing. We might say that a muscle needs to be flexible to be strong and powerful and vice versa. Watching a gymnast provides a great example of this. When performing floor work, power transfers to the upper body from the lower body and then back again. The core area needs to be very flexible but extremely strong at the same time. When a volleyball player approaches the net for a spike, the movement involves a jump with back extension and flexion at the abs when the ball is struck. This "wind up" before the strike—initiated in the core—is where much of the hitting power comes from.

HOW AND WHEN TO TRAIN THE CORE

The off-season and preseason phases of a training program are the most valuable times to prepare the body's overall strength and fitness for the more specific training that will come as the season progresses. During these two periods of training, core training should focus on high-volume drills that include a combination of stability, balance, strength, and endurance. As training progresses toward the in-season, core training should increase in intensity and become more sport-specific. Once the competitive season begins, it's time to pare down core training and focus on maintaining the strength gained. Table 5.2 highlights the various emphases of core training during the different phases of the season.

Core training should be incorporated into your program so that you reap the benefits while still meeting your other training goals for the day. You can do this by integrating core training into a warm-up or cool-down, or into the body of your program. As a warm-up, the core exercises should be less intense and geared toward the total body. This helps increase body temperature and prepares the body for more intense work. Performing the core work at the end of a program prevents fatigue setting in before an intense workout that requires the core to be fresh. For example, on a day your workout requires heavy squatting, remember that the midsection is an integral part of the supporting muscle groups for those exercises. If you do too many core exercises before the squatting workout, the trunk area may become fatigued and negatively affect the squatting workout.

Core work can also be placed within a workout, executed between strength exercises as a superset or circuit-type program. This keeps the heart rate up during the training session, but allows you to work alternate muscle groups. An especially intense or specific core workout can be enough of a day's workout by itself in some cases.

Where you place the core work within your session may also depend on what part of the training year you are in. You will want to focus more on general core work in the off-season and on core work specific to your sport during the in-season.

The core work we recommend is not limited to isolated abdominal and low back exercises. Some of the best core work includes the contraction and stabilization of several joints and muscle groups, which make the workout more sport-specific. Thus, when designing strength programs and choosing exercises, it is important to examine how several muscle groups and joints work together to create a specific movement.

Table 5.2   Off-Season, Preseason, and In-Season Emphasis on the Core

Season	Volume (sets × reps)	Intensity
Off-Season	High (12 × 25)	Low to moderate
Preseason	Moderate to high (8-12 × 10-25)	Moderate to high
In-Season	Moderate (8 × 10-15)	Moderate

DRILLS TO DEVELOP THE CORE

The core area should be trained the same way that individual muscles and muscle groups are, starting with general strength, stability, and proprioception exercises in the off-season and into the preseason. The volume of exercises is high, but the intensity and complexity of the exercises are low. As the season moves on and specific strength becomes more important, exercises become progressively more sport-specific and increase in intensity and complexity. Throughout the competitive season for your particular sport, we recommended a mix designed to meet your sport-specific goals while maintaining the strength you have gained. See the sport-specific program tables presented in chapter 9.

GENERAL STRENGTH

Low-level exercises that focus on general strength of the abdominal, low back, and hip muscles are the first step in any core-training program. These exercises are best executed using body weight as resistance. Performing an exercise without external resistance first is a great way to get a feel for the exercise and correct technique in a safe setting. Using just your body weight helps to develop the neuromuscular patterns that will allow you to complete the exercise correctly when you add resistance later. Complete each drill slowly, focusing on controlling the movement. Use a three count when performing the eccentric (muscle lengthens during contraction) and concentric (muscle shortens during contraction) portion of the exercise. Performing these drills slowly and with control prevents you from relying on momentum and compensating with other muscle groups.

ANKLE TOUCH

This exercise focuses on the abdominal muscle group, and uses the hip muscles for stabilization.

1. While lying with a flat back on the floor, position the feet flat on the floor, shoulder-width apart. The angle at the knee should be about 90 degrees. Extend the arms straight toward the feet just off the floor.

2. Using the abdominals, lift the shoulder blades off the floor while pressing the low back into the floor.

3. Repeat touches toward the feet in a controlled manner. The rectus abdominis will hold the body in position while the obliques control the dynamic motion.

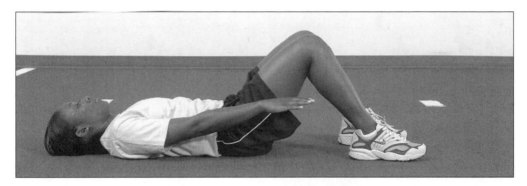

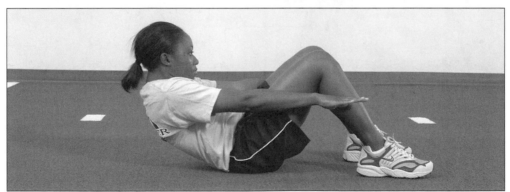

ABDOMINAL CURL

This is the traditional crunch exercise. The exercise is different from ankle touches because it uses a greater range of motion through the abdominals.

1. Lie with a flat back on the floor, knees bent and feet flat, hands behind the head, eyes looking at the ceiling.
2. Use the abdominal muscles to pull the upper body so that the shoulder blades come off the ground.
3. Don't pull the neck with the hands or allow the feet to come off the ground.

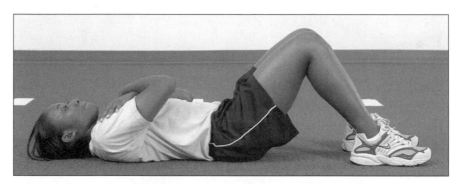

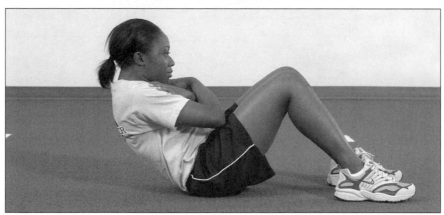

V-UP

This exercise focuses on strengthening the abdominal muscles and the hip flexors and extensors.

1. Lie with a flat back on the floor with arms extended above the head. The legs are straight out from the body so that a straight line is created from fingers to toes.
2. Initiate the movement by raising straight legs from the hips in a controlled manner. The upper body should mirror this movement as one rigid body part, forming a V with the body or bringing the hands to the feet.
3. The glutes balance the body at the top of the movement.
4. Return to the starting position slowly and in control.

V-ups can also be used to work the obliques by moving the upper body to the right and left during alternate repetitions.

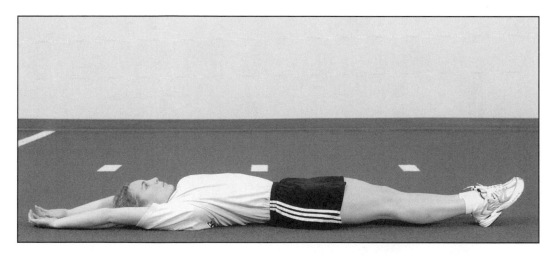

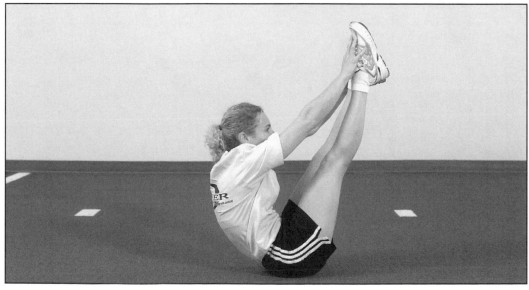

BENCH OBLIQUES

This exercise strengthens the transverse obliques of the abdominal group.

1. Begin lying on your side on a bench. A partner will hold your legs as demonstrated in the photos below.
2. Distribute your weight evenly on the hip that is on the bench.
3. Place the arms across the chest or behind the head and slowly use the obliques to raise the body in a sideways motion.
4. Return to the starting position by lowering slowly.
5. Repeat the exercise on each side.
6. Modify the exercise to include the rectus abdominis by adding a twist of the upper body toward the ceiling after the each raise.

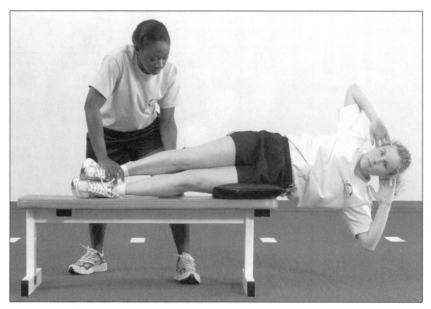

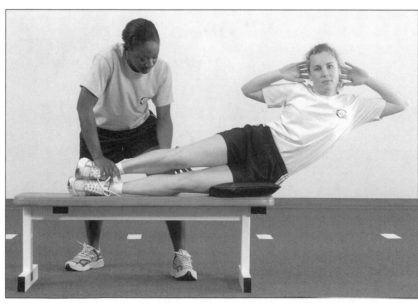

HANGING KNEE RAISE

This exercise strengthens the hip flexors and extensors, while using the abdominal group as stabilizers.

1. With the arms in straps or simply hanging by the hands from a chin-up bar, start with the body in a vertical straight line.
2. While maintaining a rigid upper body, lift the knees toward the chest, slowly and with control to prevent the body from swinging.
3. Return to the starting position.
4. Modify this exercise by lifting the lower legs straight out from the body until parallel with the floor. This makes the drill more complex and difficult to do.

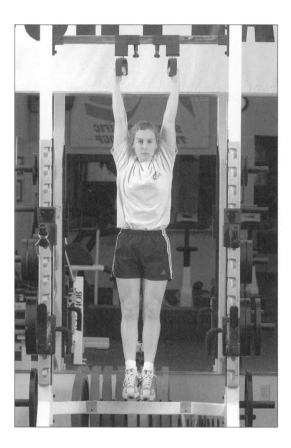 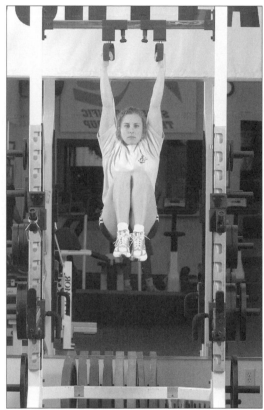

REVERSE CRUNCH

This exercise strengthens the hip extensors and flexors while using the abdominal group to stabilize.

1. While lying with a flat back on the floor, position the feet flat on the floor, shoulder-width apart. The angle at the knee should be about 90 degrees. Extend the arms straight toward the feet just off the floor.
2. Keep the back flat with the low back pressed into the ground. Keep the head on the floor and the arms resting at the sides.
3. Using the abdominal muscles and hip flexors, slowly raise the feet off the ground keeping a 90-degree angle at the knee. Lift until the hips come off the ground. This should not be a rolling movement but a lifting movement.
4. In a controlled manner, lower the feet back to the floor.

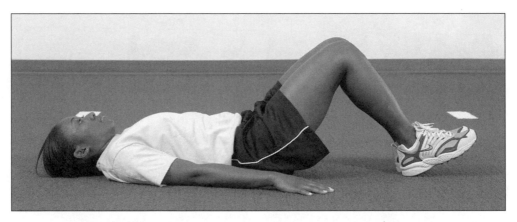

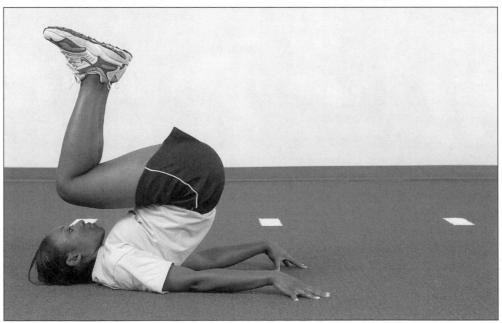

TWIST

This exercise strengthens the obliques of the abdominal group with the support of the complete abdominal group as stabilizers. You can perform twists from either a seated or a standing position.

1. The seated twists begin in the ankle-touch position (page 85, bottom photo), except that you hold a light medicine ball or weight plate.
2. Maintaining a flat back and keeping the shoulders pulled back, hold the ball or plate out from the chest.
3. Alternate twisting from right to left, bringing the ball or plate down toward the hips during each repetition. Be sure to keep the implement in front of the chest throughout the movement.
4. To modify, repeat the exercise from a standing position. Standing during this exercise may be more sport-specific for some athletes. By standing in an athletic position, with ankles, knees, and hips slightly bent and trunk stabilized, you can simulate many sport-specific movements.

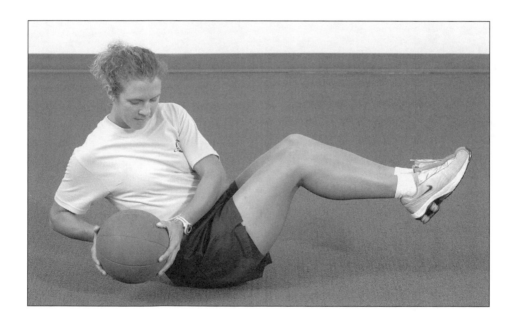

GLUTE–HAM: BENT KNEE

This exercise strengthens the erector spinae muscle of the low back and the hamstrings, with an emphasis on the gluteal muscle group. The abdominal muscle group provides stabilization. See also the glute–ham: straight leg exercise (back extension) in chapter 4 (page 71) for a complementary exercise.

1. Start in the midposition of a hyperextension on a glute–ham bench so that the upper body is in a straight line, but the knees are bent.
2. Keep the head in a neutral position and hands placed across the chest or behind the head.
3. Begin the movement by contracting the hamstrings. Focus on driving the knees into the pad and not allowing them to drop from the parallel position.
4. Continue contracting the hamstrings until the torso is perpendicular with the floor. The upper body from the knees to the head should maintain a straight line.
5. Use the abdominal muscles and low back to stabilize this position.
6. Slowly return to the starting position.

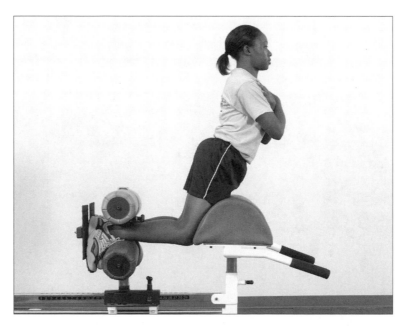

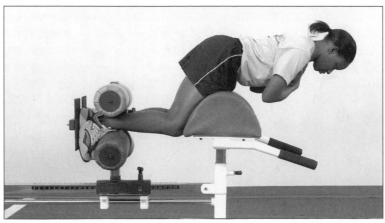

BASIC POWER

After you have mastered the general strength core exercises, you are ready to incorporate basic power core exercises. It is important to complete the exercises using correct technique before moving on to more complex movements. You'll perform these basic power exercises at higher speeds or using more resistance than simple body weight to more closely simulate sport-specific movements. This phase of training prepares the core muscles for sport-specific training.

Using medicine balls in different drills is an excellent way to develop basic power. Drills with medicine balls can be performed standing and in different directions. As the exercises engage more stabilizing muscles throughout the movement, they become more sport-specific.

MEDICINE BALL: CHEST PASS

This standing exercise promotes balance and stability. The entire body is used during this exercise, with emphasis on the upper body.

1. Start with the feet under the hips and staggered, and with ankles, knees, and hips slightly flexed. Stand four to five feet from a partner.
2. With the medicine ball at chest level and about five inches from the chest, use the arms and hands to explosively project the ball to your partner.
3. Your partner catches the ball in the same position at the chest as it was thrown.
4. Your partner immediately rebounds the medicine ball back to you.

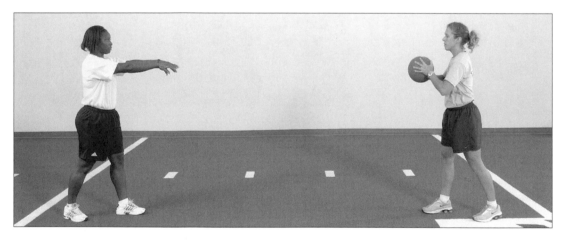

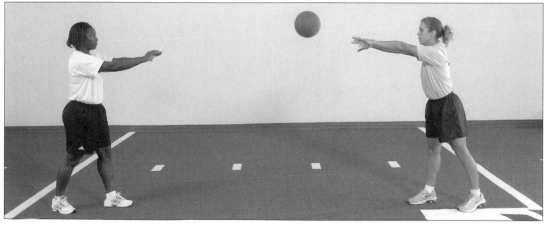

MEDICINE BALL: TWIST PASS

This standing exercise promotes balance and stability of the entire body, with emphasis on the rotation of the upper body.

1. Each partner's body position should be the same as with the chest pass, but partners face opposite directions, with direct alignment of one partner's hips with the other's. Athletes should stand two to three feet apart.

2. Using a strong twisting motion with the medicine ball in front of the abdomen, pass the ball to your partner.

3. The receiving athlete should receive the ball in front of the abdomen, twist to the other side, and then return the ball.

4. When receiving the ball it is important not to twist excessively. The rebound should be quick and explosive.

5. Athletes can also perform this exercise while seated. Sitting restricts the rotation at the torso. The position is great for sports such as rowing or kayaking where the lower body is fixed.

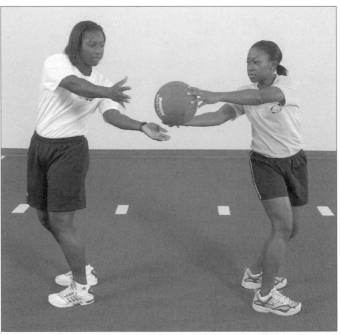

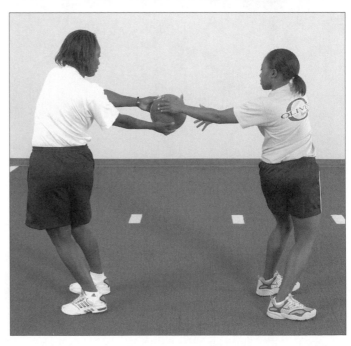

MEDICINE BALL: OVERHEAD THROW

This standing exercise promotes balance and stability of the entire body, with emphasis on the upper body.

1. Start with the feet staggered and the ankles, knees, and hips slightly flexed. Hold the medicine ball with both hands just behind the head. A partner should stand at least eight feet away.

2. Focusing on the abdominals, throw the medicine ball to the partner's chest area where she can catch it with both hands under the ball.

3. Work to throw the ball with as much power as possible while still completing the drill correctly.

4. The partner repeats the same movement.

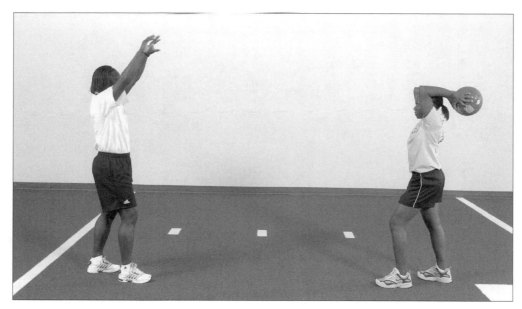

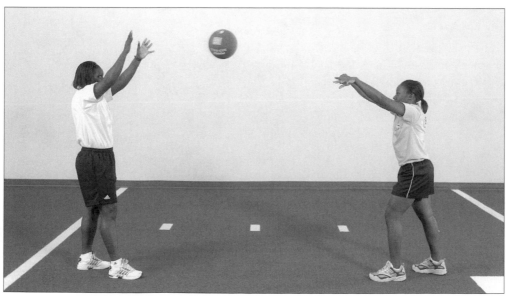

STABILITY

Stability drills can and should be implemented during the early phases of training (off-season and preseason). Whereas the general strength and basic power drills are usually dynamic, most stability drills require the athlete to hold difficult positions using the entire body, but focusing primarily on the core. Physioballs, Airex pads, Dynadiscs, and BOSU ball trainers are excellent tools to enhance the stability of the core muscles, tendons, and ligaments. These implements provide an unstable base on which the drills are executed. Some of these surfaces are very soft and some are hard and filled with air. Different surfaces create different challenges. These drills provide a change from the normal routine and can add fun to training. When performed on one leg, these drills are great for promoting single-leg balance. Single-leg balance is called upon in most court and field sports when the athlete loses balance or is pushed off balance by an opponent.

PILLARS

This exercise stabilizes the entire body but also places stress on the shoulders. The correct body position should be held for the desired amount of time for each repetition. Pillars can be performed three different ways:

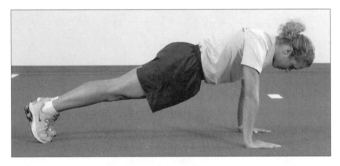

1. The first is by holding the body in a push-up position and maintaining a straight line from the head to the feet. You can modify this position for the novice by supporting the upper body on the forearms and using the elbows to hold the body weight.

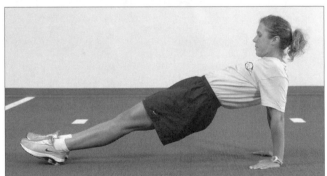

2. The second is the reverse of the first. In a faceup position, the athlete places equal weight on the hands or forearms and the feet, maintaining a straight line from the shoulders to the feet.

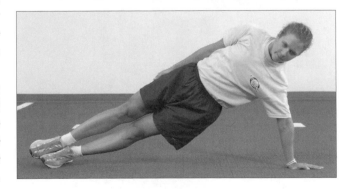

3. The last method is to maintain the position on the right and then the left side. The athlete supports her weight on one wrist or forearm and one foot. The shoulders, hips, knees, and feet should form a straight line.

BRIDGE PUSH-UP

This exercise stabilizes the entire body on the shoulders and wrists and can be done on an unstable surface. The most unstable part of the body in this exercise is the lower body.

1. Balance the feet on the ball and hold the body up with the arms on the ground in a push-up position. Keep the back flat while in this position.
2. Use the abdominals, low back, and shoulders to stabilize this position and hold for the desired amount of time.

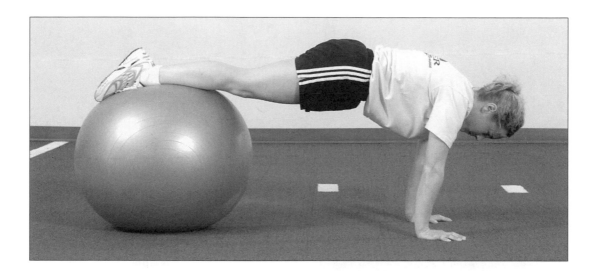

PIKE

The pike stabilizes the body on the shoulders and wrists and can be done on an unstable surface. The most unstable part of the body in this exercise is the upper body.

1. Start in the same position as for the bridge push-up. Move into a pike position by raising the hips higher than the head.
2. Return to the original position.
3. Keep the abdominal muscles and low back rigid throughout the motion.

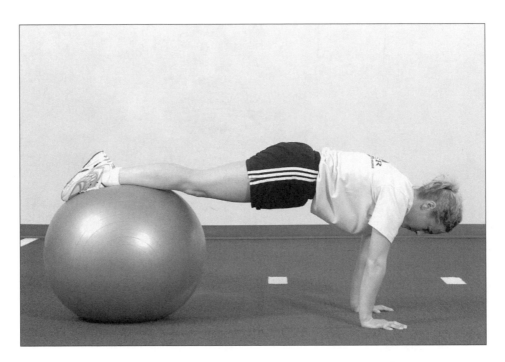

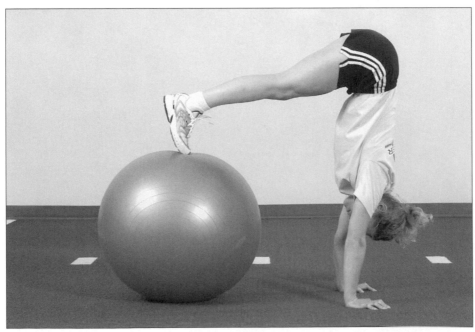

HIP HIKE

This stabilizes the entire body on the shoulders and wrists and can be done on an unstable surface. The most unstable part of the body in this exercise is the lower body.

1. Begin by lying with the back on the ground and feet on the ball.
2. Place the arms perpendicular from the body to help with balance. As you master the movement, bring the arms in toward the sides to develop greater stabilization.
3. From this position, raise the hips off the ground to create a rigid straight line from the knees to the shoulders and hold for the desired amount of time.

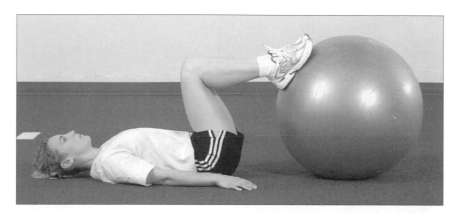

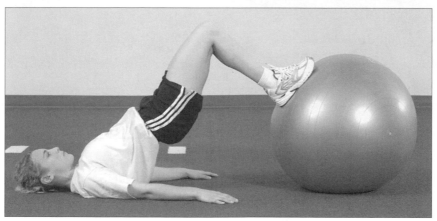

ELBOW BRIDGE

This exercise stabilizes the entire body on the shoulders and wrists and can be done on an unstable surface. The most unstable part of the body in this exercise is the upper body.

1. Using a physioball, balance the body with the toes on the ground and the elbows on the ball.
2. The body from head to toe should create a straight line.
3. Use the abdominals, low back, and shoulders to hold this rigid position for the desired amount of time.

EXTENDED CRUNCH

This drill strengthens the abdominal muscles while stabilizing with the hips and ankles.

1. Center the low back on the physioball so that you can hyperextend around the ball.
2. With hands behind the head, flex the abdominal muscles into a crunch position.
3. Slowly return back to the extended position.
4. You can modify this exercise to include the obliques by adding a twist.

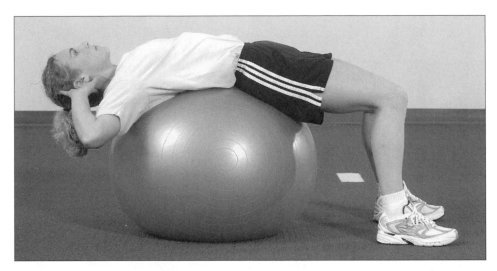

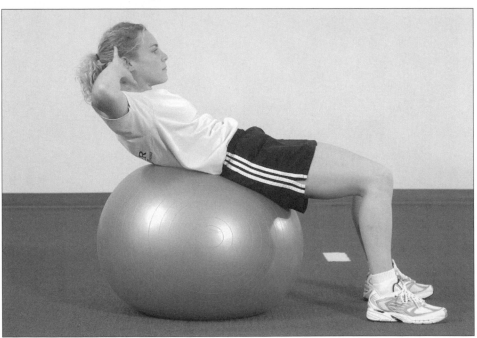

REVERSE HYPEREXTENSION

This exercise focuses on the erector spinae muscles of the low back, the hamstrings, and the gluteal muscle group. The abdominal muscle group provides stabilization.

1. Lie facedown on the physioball with the hands on the ground to help balance.
2. Using the low back muscles, gluteal muscles, and hamstrings, keep the legs straight and raise them from the ground.
3. Lower them in a slow and controlled manner to the starting position.

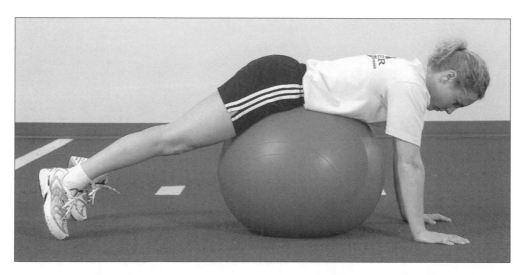

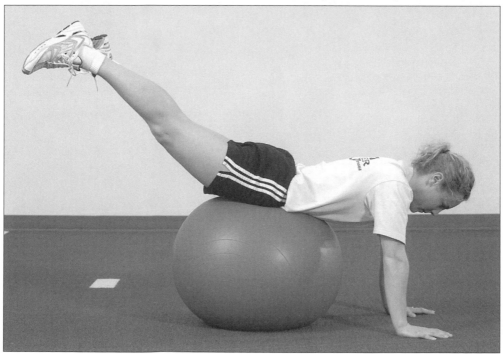

HYPEREXTENSION

This exercise focuses on the erector spinae muscles of the low back, the hamstrings, and the gluteal muscle group. The abdominal muscle group provides stabilization.

1. Lie facedown on the physioball with the toes on the ground about one foot apart to help balance.
2. With the hands behind the head, lift the upper body using the low back and glutes. Raise the torso to full extension so that a straight line runs from the head to the toes.
3. Return to the starting position slowly and with control.

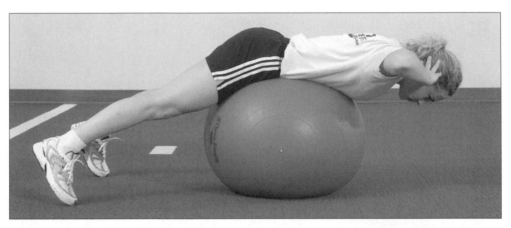

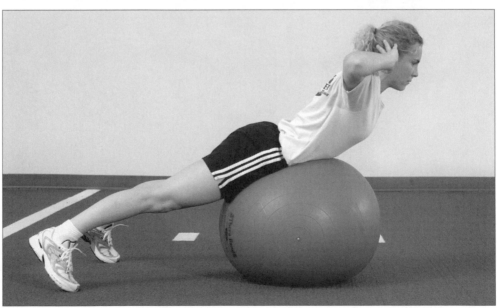

LEG CURL

This exercise strengthens the erector spinae muscles of the low back, the hamstrings, and the gluteal muscle group. The abdominal muscle group provides stabilization.

1. Begin by lying with a flat back on the ground and feet on the ball.
2. Lift the hips into the hip hike position.
3. With the feet, pull the physioball toward the gluteal muscles; feel the hamstrings contracting.
4. Use the abdominal muscles and low back to stabilize the body throughout the movement.
5. Return the physioball to its original position by slowly releasing the ball back out.
6. Remain in the hip hike position to perform repetitions of this exercise.
7. Modify the exercise by placing one foot on the physioball and holding the opposite leg in the air. This provides even more focus on the one hamstring.

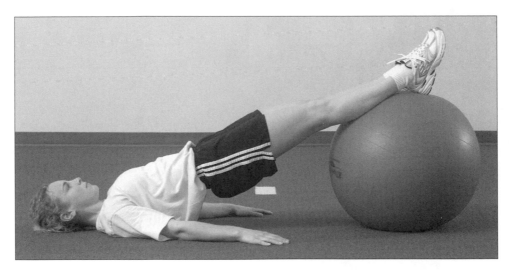

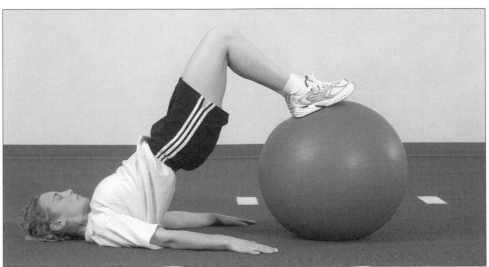

PROPRIOCEPTION AND COORDINATION

All of the stability drills just outlined can be modified and combined to enhance an athlete's proprioception and coordination. These modified or combined drills are often the most advanced and sport-specific. You must use strength, power, *and* stability while incorporating other skills at the same time. As with all exercises, you must progressively master the individual drills before combining them.

CHEST PASS ON BOSU

Follow the medicine ball chest pass drill (see page 93), but perform the passes while standing on the BOSU trainer. Pay special attention to balance and precision while throwing and catching.

SINGLE-LEG OVERHEAD THROW

Follow the instructions for the medicine ball overhead throw (see page 95), but stand on one leg or on an unstable surface such as an Airex pad or Dynadisc.

EXTENDED CRUNCH WITH PASS

Follow the instructions for the extended crunch (see page 100), but include a medicine ball overhead or chest pass to a partner. Make sure you do not use momentum from the ball to assist with abdominal flexion. First flex into a crunch, then throw the ball.

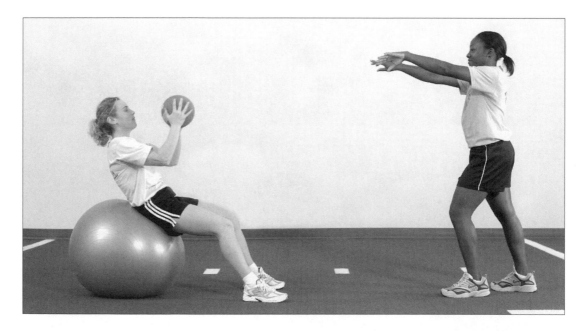

Many sport movements require a transfer of power from the lower body to the upper body, placing significant importance on the core area. The core is therefore the link during vertical, horizontal, and transverse movements. Adding core exercises to the athlete's program heightens body awareness and increases stability, strength, and coordination. This adds up to better athletic performance.

Part III
Gaining Power

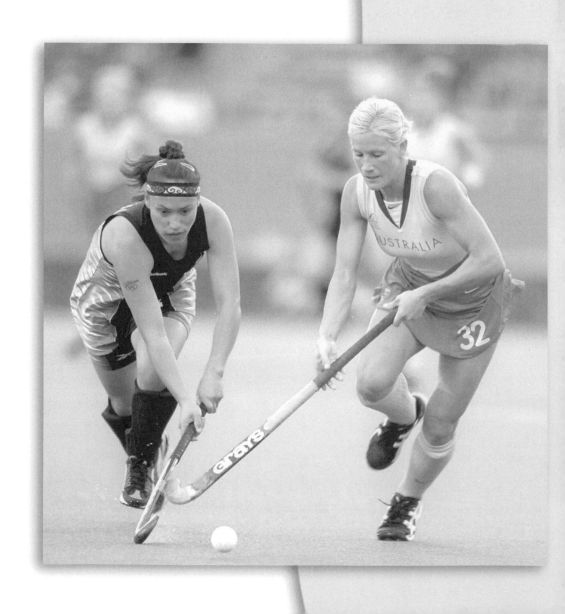

6

Strong Speed for Starting, Stopping, and Cutting

When looking at sport and the athletes that rise above the others, we often see those who are faster, stronger, and most of all more powerful. Power helps an athlete get to a loose ball first, hit a home run, finish the 100 meters strong, and explode on a last tumbling pass in gymnastics. Even in golf, a sport that has long been thought of as a finesse sport, the top performers today are the most powerful. The fact is that women are in the weight room and on the track becoming more powerful than ever in the history of women's athletics.

In part I of this book we talked about laying the foundation, a training base. You must build a strength base before incorporating an aggressive power-training program into your routine. This strength is the first component of the power formula. The second is speed. If you want to create power, you must first increase the strength and then the speed of an athlete.

Speed refers to the rate of movement from point A to point B and depends on several things. Speed coaches refer to speed in two ways. We say there is **top-end speed**—speed measured with a running start. That is, the athlete is already at full speed when she hits the start, and she is timed from that start to the designated finish. *Stride length* and power are the primary focus. The other way coaches refer to speed is by noting an athlete's **acceleration**. Acceleration is how quickly an athlete can get from a stationary position to top speed. An athlete's acceleration is measured from a stationary start. Acceleration depends on *stride frequency* (the number of times the feet push off the ground per unit of time). Testing a 40-yard (about 37 meters) dash from a stationary position is one way to measure both acceleration (stride frequency—from the start to 20 yards) and top-end speed (stride length from 20 to 40 yards). Running speed is the product of stride length and stride frequency (speed = stride length × stride frequency).

So, how is speed directly related to power? Combined with strength (maximal amount of force independent of time), speed (distance over time) is a component of power. That is, power is strength × speed. If you're missing one component, power can never be maximized.

We know that to increase power, an athlete must develop all of the physical systems of the body through specific training. It is our experience that the quickest gains in an athlete's performance, including linear speed, multidirectional speed, balance, and coordination occur by working on efficiency of movement. Technique must be the first focus for any athlete trying to improve a skill. The more efficient an athlete is technically, the less energy she expends to go faster. In this chapter we present ways athletes can improve and gain power physically and technically. Once you understand the technical aspects of running form you can practice the specific drills for starting, stopping, cutting, and shuffling. The principles for linear power (running speed) are very similar to those needed for multidirectional power. Explosive starts and efficient technical skill are essential for both. A powerful stride can be gained through a regimen that employs technical work and takes a sound approach to the physical training routine.

> Training for me is confidence. Training for me is about getting the extra edge. It is not just about running and running and running . . . it is about doing the little technical things that make me sharper, quicker, stronger and more explosive. As I have gotten older, I have learned that if I just work for work's sake, I will run myself into the ground. I now structure my training around quality, rather than quantity. Yes, age-old wisdom, but hard to implement when you are used to running yourself into the ground!
>
> *Julie Foudy, member of the 1996 and 2004 Olympic gold medal soccer teams and the 1999 World Cup Championship soccer team*

Proper technique is achieved by training the nervous system. Motor learning and muscle memory should be the first things a coach considers when setting up a training plan. The training must be sport-specific so that the drills develop the correct neuromuscular patterns. Technique training is composed of two important components:

- **Rhythm** is performing a skill with coordination and timing without considering the rate at which a skill is performed. Rhythm is achieved when a skill is done properly.
- **Tempo** is the rate at which a skill is performed.

An athlete must first have rhythm before improving tempo. A skill can't be performed correctly at a high rate of speed without first developing the muscle memory. This is important because our primary goal in training is to develop power. An elite athlete can generate maximal power because she can perform skills at a high speed. By becoming technically efficient, an athlete opens the pathways to create speed. Coupled with the strength gained in the weight room, speed helps create maximal power. In speed and power training, one of the best ways to improve rhythm and timing is by performing drills that develop your stride length.

DEVELOPING STRIDE LENGTH AND POWER

Balance, coordination, and muscle memory enable an athlete to generate maximal power against the running surface. Coaches and athletes must first understand the primary muscle group used in sprinting—the hamstrings. Check out the hamstrings of any world-class sprinter. When the hamstrings contract during a sprint, they create a pulling motion. Think of sprinting as pulling the running surface past the body. To do this effectively you must follow these guidelines.

- Maintain a tall posture with a slight forward body lean.

- Work the arms in opposition to the legs in a chin-to-pocket pattern with elbows bent at 90 degrees and arm rotation coming from the shoulders.

- Make sure the thigh is parallel to the running surface during the active phase of the stride.

- Ensure that the ball (front half) of the foot contacts the ground on the downsweep of the leg.

- The foot should contact the ground when it is below the knee, not ahead of it.

- The foot on the ground pulls past the body and toes off.

- At toeoff, the heel sweeps upward toward the gluteals during the recovery.

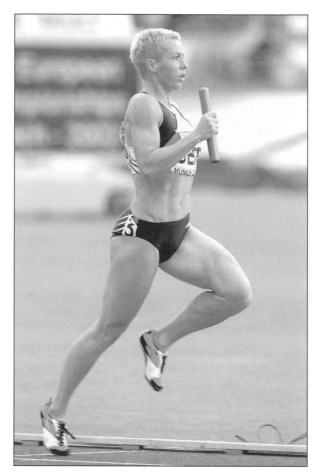

Well-developed hamstrings and proper technique combine to produce powerful sprinting.

As a general rule, when running forward, backward, or sideways, the point where your foot contacts the ground should be directly below the knee. Sometimes you hear coaches say, "Keep your feet under you." The technical term coaches may use is *shin angles*. A positive shin angle occurs when the ball (front half) of the athlete's foot lands in the front of the knee. This heel-toe running is used by distance runners and is important for shock absorption but not good for sprinting. A neutral shin angle occurs when the tibia (lower leg) lands perpendicular to the ground, and a negative shin angle occurs when the ball of the foot lands slightly behind the front of the knee. Negative and neutral shin angles are favored in sports that involve short sprints and change of direction. The athlete's weight is on the front of the foot, which allows quicker turnover (stride frequency) and acceleration.

From this description you can see how complex the movement pattern for a sprint is. Breaks in correct technique will cost an athlete overall speed. This is why running technique drills are so important. To generate an explosive stride an athlete must have sufficient strength to control her body movements.

Table 6.1 provides a running evaluation form that coaches can use to assess an athlete's running form and uncover weaknesses they may want to work to improve through drills.

Here are five exercises that we consider very effective for improving stride and leg power for many sports. Refer to the final chapter on sport-specific programs for a detailed program that incorporates these five exercises in a manner that is appropriate for your sport.

Table 6.1 Running Evaluation Form

Athlete	Start	Arm action	Knee lift	Toe-off	Heel action	Body position	Lateral swaying	Comments

From *Athletic Strength for Women* by David Oliver and Dana Healy, 2005, Champaign, IL: Human Kinetics.

WALKING LUNGE

The walking lunge is one of our favorites. This exercise should be incorporated into most athletes' regimens. It helps to develop athletic strength in the gluteals, hamstrings, hip flexors, and quadriceps and is performed through a full range of motion. The walking lunge is detailed in chapter 4 (see page 72).

POWER SKIP

The power skip is an exaggerated version of the high-knee skip presented in chapter 8. However, you will spend more time in the air and use a more pronounced arm action in this exercise. The movement follows a hop-step sequence.

1. Perform a skipping movement (hop step) by alternately driving the right and left knees upward.
2. Explode off the ground, getting as much airtime as possible, but remaining in control.
3. Aggressively swing the arms from the shoulders.
4. Contact the ground on the ball of the foot maintaining a stable ankle position.
5. Repeat the power skip on the opposite side for the prescribed number of repetitions.
6. The movements should be rhythmic and controlled.

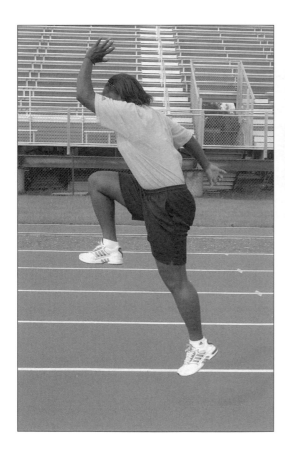 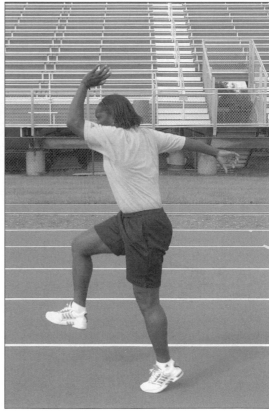

BARRIER STRIDES

This is one of the best drills for learning how to stride. It is also an excellent way to make the transition from power skips to bounding. For this drill you need a tape measure and eight foam barriers six inches (15 centimeters) high. If you don't have foam, use a material that will not hurt you if you land on it. You may also use minihurdles; however, these can break when hit. This drill is appropriate for athletes who have a good strength base. The settings below are designed for varsity-level high school athletes and advanced athletes.

1. Set up eight barriers, each five feet (one and a half meters) apart.
2. Run to and stride over each of the eight barriers.
3. Stride so that the thighs are parallel to the ground. The arms should move in a chin-to-pocket arc, and the foot contacts should be on the balls of the feet with a stable, locked ankle. Maintain a slight forward body lean.
4. Increase the distance between barriers to six feet (1.8 meters), then seven (2.1 meters), and so forth. When technique breaks down, stop.
5. Perform three repetitions for each distance.

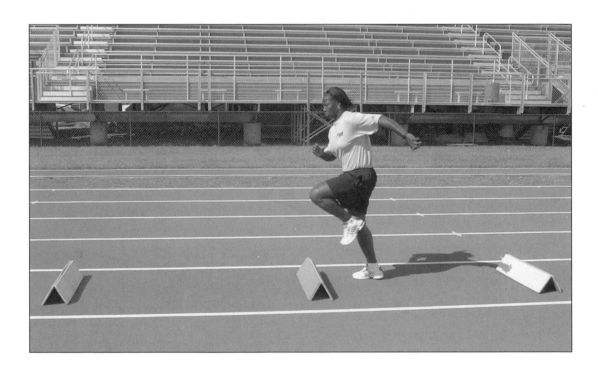

BOUNDING

Bounding is an overexaggeration of the stride. To bound properly the athlete must bring her knees up so that the thigh is parallel to the ground, then pull the heel toward the hamstring. The arm action is also long and exaggerated. The explosive nature of this exercise occurs during the ground contact, or landing phase, and the takeoff phase, where a tremendous amount of strength and balance must be exhibited. To perform the drill correctly, the athlete must explode with aggressive arm action and leg drive on takeoff.

1. Take several running approach steps into the bound.
2. The initial movement is an aggressive, explosive drive off the back leg, with the opposite knee driving forward at the same time. The heel of the front leg should remain directly below the knee, and the thigh should be parallel to the ground. You will leave the ground while bounding forward. Maintain an aggressive chin-to-pocket arm action.
3. Aggressively contact the surface with the ball of the front foot, keeping the ankle locked and stable.
4. Repeat the movement on the opposite side.

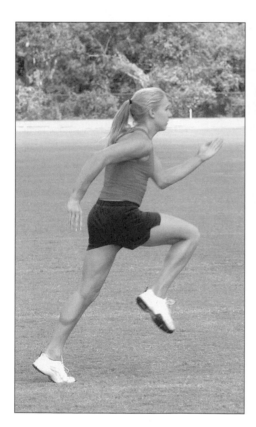
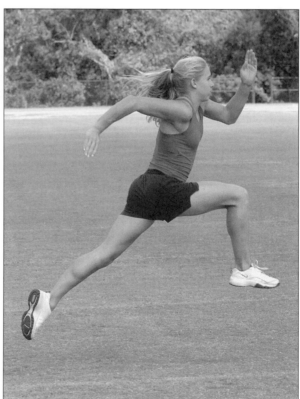

WEIGHTED SLED TOWING

Towing a sled is an excellent way to increase the intensity of running. An athlete greatly increases the force of each stride in this form of training.

1. Place weights on a tow sled. The amount of weight depends on your goal. Less weight will allow you to pull the sled faster and maintain a more accurate running technique. Heavier weights will improve your overall strength but may compromise technique. It is good practice to start your training with lighter weights. Do two to three workouts with a weight you can tow comfortably. You can then adjust the weight based on your goal. If you are in the off-season working on endurance, you might tow a light weight 10 × 80 yards or meters. But if you are in a preseason mode, increase the weight and perform 15 × 30 to 50 yards or meters.

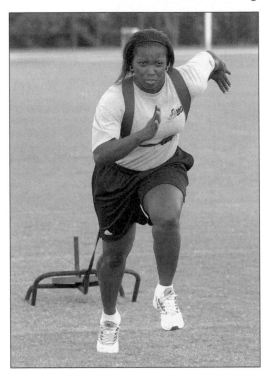

2. Place the tow harness on the upper body.
3. Run for the designated distance concentrating on explosive leg drive, aggressive arm action, and proper running technique.
4. Stay low as you drive forward.

DEVELOPING STRIDE FREQUENCY

Stride frequency is as important to obtaining a powerful running stride as stride length is. When developing stride frequency the primary goal is to develop muscle memory. Stride frequency is gained when muscles fire rapidly in a rhythmic fashion. Stride frequency training focuses on performing the following exercises as efficiently as possible and as rapidly as possible. You want to develop the neural pathways that allow for rapid firing of muscles.

Although the primary sprinting muscles are the hamstrings, you must consider the hip flexors when training for stride frequency. The hip flexors are responsible for the recovery phase of the stride—pulling the heel through and elevating the leg at the hip joint. This can also be considered as the loading or cocking phase of the sprint, so the faster you can train these muscles to load for the next stride, the faster you can become. Training the hip flexors through stride-frequency work will increase your speed dramatically.

TWO-FOOT BARRIER STRIDES

This drill incorporates classic high-knee form running. Using a six-inch barrier will force you to keep your knees high. This barrier drill is best done before the barrier strides (see page 112), with one foot between each barrier so that you are working both stride frequency and stride length.

1. Set up eight foam barriers six inches (15 centimeters) high and five feet (one and a half meters) apart.

2. Run over each barrier, taking two steps between each. Focus on rapid ground contact and arm action as you run through the barriers.

3. Maintain proper running technique with the thighs parallel to the ground, chin-to-pocket arm action, and foot contact on the balls of the feet.

4. Increase the distance between the barriers by one foot (.3 meters) after three reps.

BUNGEE SPRINTS

This is an advanced exercise that requires a significant amount of strength and balance. Make sure the running surface is flat, and do not overstretch the bungee cord. Overspeed training is a training modality that uses supramax (more than max) running to affect the neural and muscular systems. When nerves and muscles are overloaded in this way, they respond by adapting to the training stress and making the athlete more powerful.

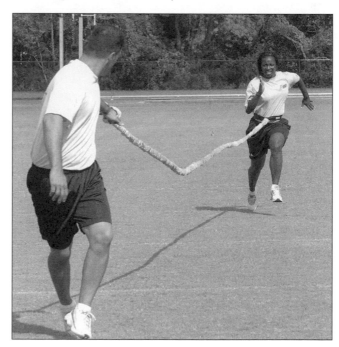

1. Use a 12- to 15-foot (four- to four and a half- meters) bungee cord with a safety cover. Loop one end of the bungee cord around the waist. A partner holds the opposite end and stands 20 to 30 yards or meters in front of you so that the cord is taut.

2. When you start running toward the partner, the bungee cord will create a slingshot effect enabling you to turn your legs over at a greater rate than you are normally capable of.

3. Maintain proper technique, and run the full distance of 20 to 30 yards or meters.

DOWNHILL RUNNING

Athletes and coaches have used downhill running for many years as an overspeed training method. An added benefit is that athletes must eccentrically load the muscles of the lower extremity to maintain balance. Stimulating the nerves and muscles in this way may decrease the number of injuries that female athletes sustain during eccentric loading in game situations.

1. Position yourself at the top of a gradual hill 20 to 30 yards or meters long.
2. Run as fast as you can down the hill while maintaining proper technique. Keep your body perpendicular to the running surface while maintaining a foot strike on the balls of your feet.
3. When you reach the bottom of the hill decelerate slowly (don't put on the brakes).
4. Repeat for the designated number of repetitions.

SLIDE BOARD SPRINTS

Slide board sprints are great for developing the hip flexor muscles, which are important for elevating the leg at the hip and increasing stride frequency.

1. Using a slide board and foot covers, position yourself in a track start.
2. Sprint for two to four sets of 30 seconds. The feet should slide and not leave the board.
3. Keep the back flat and make sure the legs go through a full range of motion.

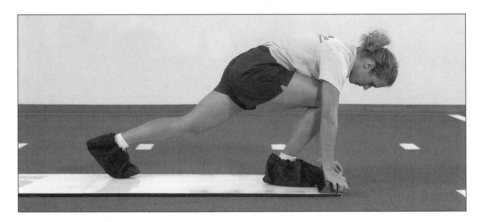

STOPPING

A chapter on explosive running for sports would not be complete without talking about the deceleration phase of the movement. We know that the greatest number of injuries occur when an athlete stops, plants, or decelerates suddenly. Muscle strains and ligament tears, especially in the knee and other parts of the lower extremity, are the most common injuries caused by these actions. Working on drills specific to the deceleration phase of running will help prevent these injuries and lead to better performance. The following drills teach you how to stop quickly and safely.

STOP-AND-GO DRILL

You can perform this drill on a court or field. Wear proper athletic-specific footwear for your sport and for the terrain. Cleats are appropriate for field training. You need three or four cones set up 10 to 15 yards or meters apart in a straight line. The distance between cones depends on whether short or long sprints are most appropriate for your sport.

1. Starting at the first cone, accelerate toward the next.
2. When you are two to three yards from the cone, decelerate with rapid steps.
3. Stop at the cone with the right foot forward and in an athletic body position, keeping the knees bent, chest forward slightly, and hips down so that you are using your whole body to stop, not just your legs. Pause for two to three seconds after each step so that you have adequate time to reset your feet. Accelerate toward the next cone.
4. Perform this drill leading with the same foot on the stop for all the cones.
5. Repeat the drill leading with the opposite foot.

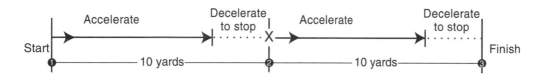

DIAGONAL SKATING

This is an excellent drill for all sports and helps to develop lower-extremity power, endurance, and stability. For training strength and endurance, the athlete performs this drill by walking in the skating position. For power, the athlete performs a diagonal leap in a skating motion.

1. From a standing position explode to the front right (diagonal movement) off the left foot and land on the right in a stable and controlled position.
2. Upon landing get as low as you can while maintaining balance.
3. Come out of the position and explode off the right leg moving in a diagonal pattern.
4. Keep the chest forward (not beyond the front leg on landing) and the back flat. The body will be in a compact position.

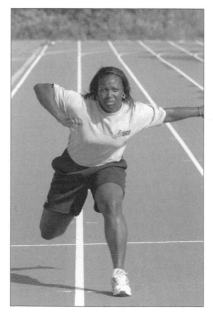
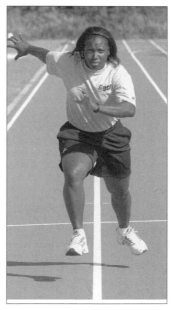

AGILITY: CHANGE OF DIRECTION

Multidirectional speed, often called agility, incorporates many of the same principles as linear speed. To maintain speed when changing direction you want to stay in an athletic position with the knees and hips bent, the chest slightly forward, and the back flat. You want to move on the balls of your feet with aggressive arm action. All movements should be rhythmic. With change-of-direction training, you must focus on quick feet during deceleration, just like you drill quick feet when accelerating. Change-of-direction drills improve performance and reduce the risk of injury.

CUTTING DRILL

Many coaches and athletes assume that cutting is something you do only as needed in a game or competitive situation. Actually cutting is a skill like any other and can and should be trained. Women who are not adept in cutting and who change direction inefficiently are prone to injury. This drill can be done as a warm-up or at full speed. When the muscular and nervous systems are fresh, this drill develops muscle memory.

1. Set up 8 to 10 cones, with each cone two to four yards or meters apart in a zig-zag pattern as shown in the figure. Adjust the cone distance based on how quickly you want to change direction.
2. Start at cone 1. Sprint under control (60 to 70 percent effort) to cone 2.
3. Decelerate just before reaching cone 2 by taking quick, short steps.
4. Pass cone 2 and make a left-footed cut. When cutting stay in a low, athletic position so that you remain balanced and under control.
5. Drive off the left foot so that the hips turn and face the next cone.
6. Accelerate to the next cone (this time making a right-footed cut and driving off the right foot) and continue the drill in the same fashion until you have cut off of all the cones.

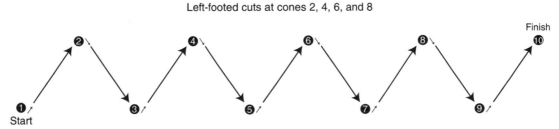

Left-footed cuts at cones 2, 4, 6, and 8

Right-footed cuts at cones 3, 5, 7, and 9

I-DRILL

This drill incorporates change-of-direction patterns. It can be performed indoors on a court or on a field. The focus is on acceleration, deceleration, and cutting. Set up three cones 5 to 10 yards apart in a straight line. At the end cones, mark a short line perpendicular to the line formed by the cones.

1. Assume an athletic position with the feet directly below the hips and face cone 1.
2. Shuffle to cone 2 and plant the right foot while touching the short line near the cone.
3. Turn, and sprint to cone 3. Decelerate with quick steps, and plant the left foot as you touch the line near cone 3.
4. Shuffle to cone 1 to finish the drill.

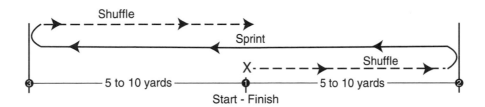

SHUTTLE DRILL

Shuttles are excellent for training and for testing. Athletes who cut efficiently will perform well on this exercise (see also chapter 2 for a shuttle test). This drill may be done individually or in groups of five. For teams, set up five groups of three cones each 5 yards or meters apart, as shown in the figure below. Five athletes will start on cone 1 and race.

1. Start facing cone 1. On the go signal, turn and sprint to cone 2.
2. Decelerate and plant the right foot on the line at cone 2. Touch the hand to the line. Make sure the body is in a good athletic position and under control.
3. Accelerate off cone 2 and sprint to cone 3. Decelerate, cut off the left foot, and touch the line.
4. Finish by sprinting through cone 1.

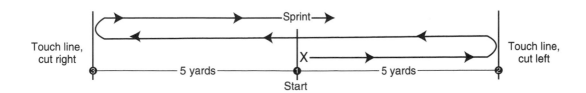

STAR DRILL

Use five 12-inch (about 30 centimeter) cones for this drill. From a center point (X in illustration below), arrange cones three to five yards or meters out to form a circle. An imaginary line connecting the cones in sequence forms a star (see figure). Vary the distance between the center and the perimeter cones depending on your sport. If you want to emphasize quickness, place the cones three yards from the center; if you are more interested in drilling top-speed change of direction, place the cones five yards from the center.

1. Start at the center cone.
2. On the go command sprint to cone 1, make a left-footed cut and knock the cone over, then sprint to cones 2, 3, 4, and 5 in sequence, making left-footed cuts for each. As you cut at each subsequent cone, knock it over until all are knocked down.
3. The drill is over when the athlete runs past cone 5.
4. The following are variations of the star drill:
   - All left-footed cuts
   - All right-footed cuts
   - Shuffle only

You can complete this drill one athlete at a time or in small groups by setting up three to five stations of five cones and dividing into teams of three, for example. On a whistle all five athletes will knock over all five cones. The first athlete to knock over the fifth cone wins. Performing the star drill is a fun way to train.

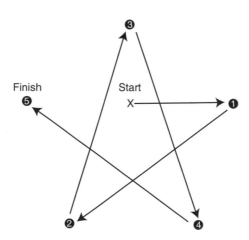

Table 6.2 provides a six-week speed training program. This program is designed for the preseason when an athlete is getting ready for competition. Although you may use some of these exercises in your off-season, remember the periodization model discussed in chapter 1. As the competitive season nears, the intensity of work increases and the volume decreases. Thus you'll want to include most of your speed and agility training, which is high intensity, only after you have established a solid base of strength and endurance through off-season training. However, if toward the end of your off-season, you wish to start including speed training, simply reduce the

Table 6.2 Preseason Speed and Agility Training

Week	1		2		3		4		5		6	
Day	1	2	1	2	1	2	1	2	1	2	1	2
Stride length	Choose 2		Choose 2		Choose 2		Choose 2		Choose 2		Choose 2	
Bounding		3 × 6		3 × 6		3 × 6		3 × 8		3 × 8		3 × 8
Stride frequency	Choose 2		Choose 2		Choose 2		Choose 2		Choose 2		Choose 2	
Downhill running		8 × 25 yd		8 × 25 yd		8 × 25 yd		8 × 25 yd		6 × 30 yd		6 × 30 yd
Deceleration	Choose 1 or 2		Choose 1		Choose 1		Choose 1		Choose 1		Choose 1	
Bungee sprints or weighted sled towing		4 × 30 yd		4 × 30 yd		4 × 30 yd		4 × 30 yd		4 × 35 yd		4 × 35 yd
Agility	Choose 1		Choose 1 or 2		Choose 1 or 2		Choose 1 or 2		Choose 1 or 2		Choose 1 or 2	
Slide board sprints		3 × 30 sec		3 × 30 sec		4 × 30 sec		4 × 30 sec		6 × 15 sec		6 × 15 sec
Advanced*	Choose 1		Choose 1		Choose 1		Choose 1		Choose 1		Choose 1	

Stride length	Sets × reps	Level of difficulty
Barrier strides (1 foot)	6 × 8 barriers 5 ft, 6 ft, 7 ft	Moderate
Power skip	4 × 8 contacts	Moderate
Bounding	4 × 4-6 contacts	Moderate to advanced
Weighted sled towing	4 × 30-40 yd	Moderate to advanced

Stride frequency	Sets × reps	Level of difficulty
Barrier strides (2 feet)	6 × 8 barriers 5 ft, 6 ft, 7 ft	Low to moderate
Downhill running	8 × 25-30 yd	Moderate
Slide board sprints	4 × 30 sec	Moderate
Cycle hops	4 × 4 hops	Advanced
Bungee sprints	4 × 30-35 yd	Advanced

Deceleration	Sets × reps	Level of difficulty
Skating (walk)	4 × 20 steps	Low to moderate
Skating (bound)	4 × 10 diagonal bounds	Moderate
Stop-and-go drill	5 × 10 cones, 10 yds apart	Moderate

Agility	Sets × reps	Level of difficulty
I-drill	1 × 5	Moderate
Cutting drill	4 × 10 cones	Low to moderate
Shuttle drill	1 × 4-6	Moderate
Star drill	1 × 4-6	Moderate

*Advanced drills are noted in the level of difficulty column.

1 inch = 2.54 centimeters; 1 foot = 0.3048 meters; 1 yard = 0.9144 meters

number of sets or reps or perform them only one day a week rather than the two days you would during the preseason.

Before performing an explosive running program, you must warm up thoroughly. Chapter 8 explains how to devise a proper warm-up. To prepare yourself for the speed drills in this chapter, you must include quickness movements in your warm-up. In particular, you should begin this program with two sets of 6 × 20 yards or meters of each of the following warm-up drills:

High-knee skip
Heel kick
Straight-leg toe touch
Carioca
Fast-feet backpedal

Follow these with two sets of four fast-feet drills (see pages 162 to 163). After a thorough warm-up, you will be ready complete a strong speed workout.

7

Explosiveness for Jumping, Running, Throwing, and Striking

Almost every athlete would like to improve the height of her vertical leap or increase the explosiveness of her jumps. Power is essential for every sport. Using power to block shots in basketball, get height on vaults in gymnastics, and spike a volleyball improves your chance of a winning performance. Plyometrics have become an effective and popular method for improving an athlete's lower- and upper-body power. Plyometrics are movements such as jumps, leaps, bounds, skips, or throws performed at a very high rate of speed and are therefore considered an advanced form of training. While most movements in traditional strength training are performed with slow, controlled movements, the explosive movements of plyometrics require balance, timing, rhythm, and muscle control and, therefore, more closely simulate the skills performed in your sport.

Power is an athlete's ability to move a mass a given distance in the least amount of time (strength × speed). Therefore, power movements are explosive and require speed. Because of the advanced nature of plyometric and explosiveness training, athletes should have a solid strength base before performing plyometric drills.

In strength training exercises such as the squat (see chapter 4, pages 65-66), the primary focus is on exerting force against a resistance for a given number of repetitions. The speed of the movement is not a factor. We actually want athletes to perform a strength routine slowly while maintaining control. However, in Olympic lifts (such as the power clean) and plyometrics (such as a box hop), the focus is on the speed of the muscles' contractions while exerting force. Olympic lifts and plyometric drills can also simulate many of the movements performed in competition. For example, bounding drills are an advanced form of running, and box shuffles simulate cutting. Recent research also suggests that correctly performing eccentric loading (plyometrics) exercises can reduce a female athlete's risk for injury. The neural changes that occur can significantly improve balance, coordination, and an athlete's overall ability to absorb ground force.

To begin building power and explosiveness, it is essential to master several movements. Then you can adapt these movements as you move into the power development training phase. One of the best ways to train for power and explosiveness is to jump rope.

Jumping rope may appear to be a simple exercise, but adding a few technical movements turns it into one of the best drills for developing coordination, speed, and timing for any sport. Each drill in this chapter can be modified depending on the goal of the exercise. For example, a more technical drill may be best completed at shorter intervals to stimulate coordination and speed. These drills are usually done for 30 seconds to one minute. Simple drills can be done as a conditioning exercise and can be done for longer periods of three, five, or even ten minutes. You can add variety to jumping rope with several variations:

- Forward jumping is a basic bounce step.
- Single-leg jumping is the basic bounce step on one leg.
- Side-to-side jumping is the basic bounce step moving laterally three to five inches left and right.
- Scissor jumping is the basic bounce step alternating feet into a forward and back movement.
- Backward jumping is the basic bounce movement while swinging the rope backward.
- Running forward requires moving quickly in a straight line while jumping rope. This is a great way to teach bounding.
- X jumps alternate a wide straddle position with a crossed-feet position.
- Double jumps require the athlete to jump higher and swing the rope faster while turning the rope twice under each single jump.

OLYMPIC WEIGHTLIFTING MOVEMENTS

Learning the Olympic lifts takes focus, time, and patience. A progression is commonly used to teach these complex movements. Developing proper technique is important. The quality of the movement always supercedes volume or intensity. Building a base of strength through the exercises in chapters 3, 4, and 5 will help prepare your body for these explosive lifts.

POWER SHRUG

Power shrugs are excellent for developing the trapezius muscle. They also form a building block for developing proper hang and power clean technique. Sports like basketball and volleyball that require explosive elevation of the scapula can benefit from this exercise.

1. The movement begins with feet in a neutral position with the weight evenly distributed on the feet throughout the motion. Slightly bend the knees so that they aren't locked. This bending will result in slight flexing at the hips. Keep the back flat. Pulling the shoulders back and keeping the head in a forward, neutral position will help hold this position throughout the movement.
2. Hold a barbell close to the body with a grip of about shoulder width.
3. Initiate the movement by extending the hips, knees, and ankles rapidly, followed immediately by an explosive shrug of the shoulders. The line of the body should not hyperextend, but form a straight vertical line from toes to head.
4. Immediately return to the starting position.

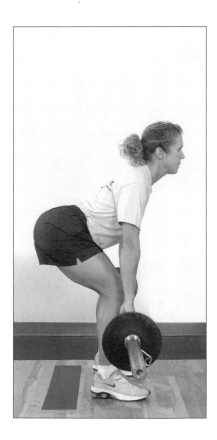
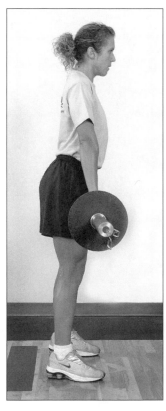
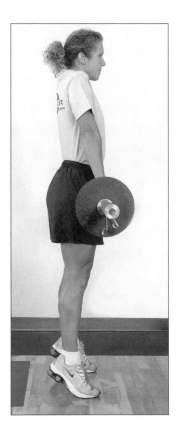

HIGH PULL

The high pull is an excellent exercise for developing proper power clean technique. It is also an excellent lift for athletes involved in jumping sports because the athlete must apply explosive force to the ground to complete the lift properly.

1. As with the power shrug, this movement begins with the feet in a neutral position with the weight evenly distributed on the feet throughout the motion. Slightly bend the knees and hips, keeping the back flat. Pulling the shoulders back and keeping the head in a forward, neutral position will help hold this position throughout the movement.

2. Hold a barbell close to the body with a grip of about shoulder width (start in the hang clean position).

3. Initiate the movement by extending the hips, knees, and ankles rapidly, followed immediately by an explosive shrug of the shoulders. The line of the body should not hyperextend, but form a straight vertical line from toes to head.

4. Immediately following the shrug, rapidly pull the bar in an upright-row motion. It should appear that the shrug and pull happen simultaneously. During technique training, the shoulders will probably do most of the pulling. When you become more proficient, the explosive extension of the ankles, knees, and hips, in addition to the shrug of the bar, will produce momentum. This momentum helps lift the bar toward the chest.

5. Immediately let the bar drop to the initial starting position.

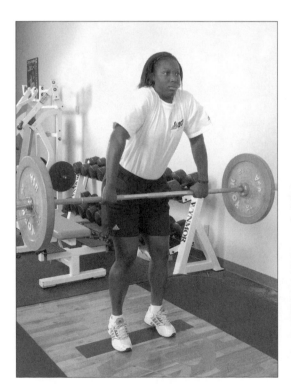
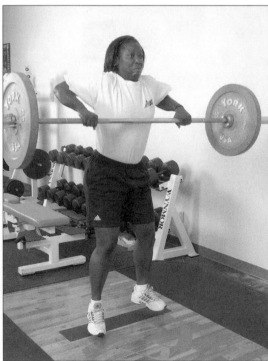

HANG CLEAN

Building on the high pull, the athlete can focus on adding the next step, the catch.

1. Follow steps one through four for the high pull to initiate the hang clean.
2. During the pull, momentum has helped pull the bar toward the chest. At this time, while keeping the bar close to the body, whip the barbell around and finish in a front-squat gripping position.
3. Simultaneously, the rest of the body should drop slightly when you flex the ankles, knees, and hips. This returns you to the starting point, but this time with the bar on the deltoids rather than hanging above the knees. Front-squat technique (page 64) greatly assists in developing strong, clean technique.

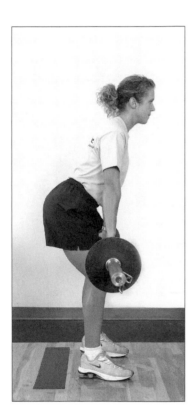
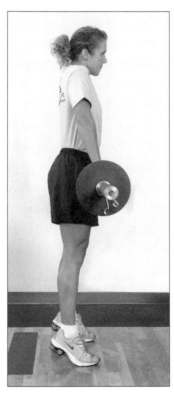
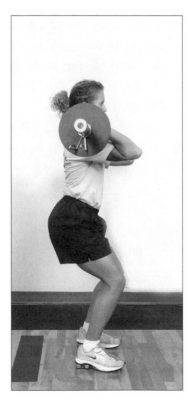

HIGH PULL FROM THE FLOOR

The high pull from the floor combines the deadlift and the high pull described earlier. These two movements must be mastered separately before they can be combined.

1. Place the feet about hip-width apart.

2. Stabilize the muscles of the core, pull back the shoulders, and keep the head in a neutral position as you lower the body as if sitting in a chair. If at any time during this movement the low back starts to round or the shoulders to fall forward, stop the exercise and work on more flexibility in the shoulders, wrists, and Achilles area as well as on strength in the torso and core before continuing.

3. With the arms relaxed and elbows rotated out to the sides, grip the bar.

4. Place your weight on the back third of the feet. Keep the entire foot in contact with the floor throughout the movement.

5. Lifting the bar begins with extension at the hip. The knees and ankles follow. Keep the chest forward with the shoulders pulled back.

6. Lift the bar until the body is in a straight, upright position.

7. As the bar passes the knees during extensions, extending the hips and the shrug cause the rapid pull of the bar.

8. Reverse the movement to bring the bar back to the ground. Keep the back rigid, and focus on the movement of the hips throughout this lift.

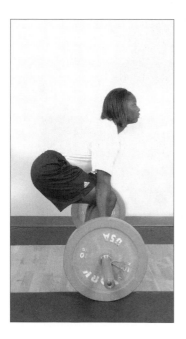 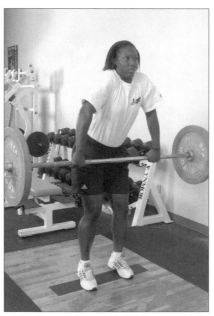 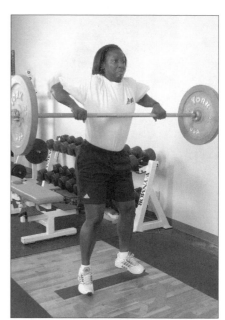

POWER CLEAN

The power clean is a modified version of the hang clean. Because this exercise requires the athlete to pull the bar from the floor, it combines complex movements, flexibility, and power.

1. The movement starts the same as a traditional deadlift. The athlete pulls the bar from the floor keeping the back flat and head forward.
2. As the bar passes the knees, the explosive movement of the hang clean begins.
3. There should be very little hesitation between these two movements. The deadlift provides upward momentum. This kick starts the next phase of the movement.
4. The exercise is finished once the bar is caught on the shoulders and the body is in a stable position.
5. Drop the bar to the floor by tipping the upper body forward and letting go of the bar.

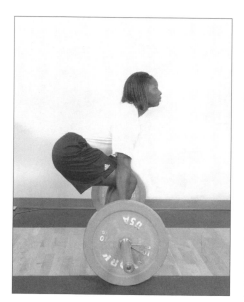 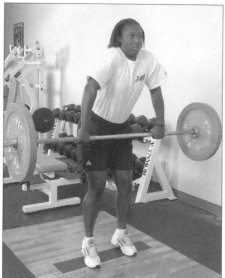

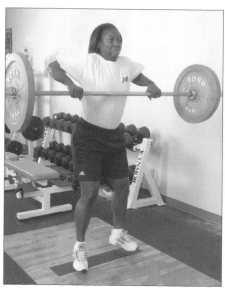 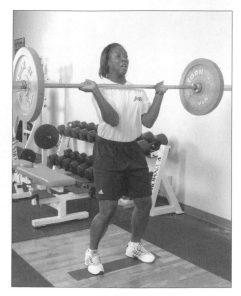

PUSH PRESS

The push press teaches an athlete to feel the power as it is transferred from the larger muscles in the lower body through the core to the smaller muscles in the upper body.

1. Begin with the barbell on the deltoids as you would if starting a front-squat movement. The abdominals and low back should remain rigid throughout the movement. The back should not hyperextend.
2. Initiate movement at the hips, knees, and ankles first with a short dip that mimics the first movement of the front squat.
3. Rapidly drive and extend the hips to produce the power that helps lift the bar from the shoulders to overhead. This movement is often referred to as a cheated military press.
4. Lower the bar slowly and carefully to the starting position.

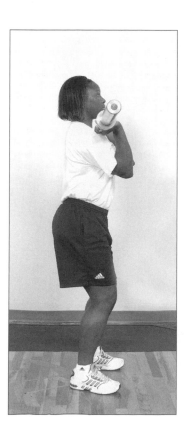 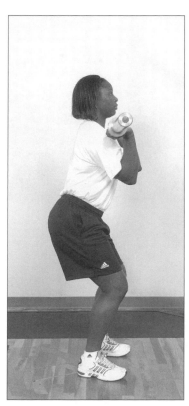 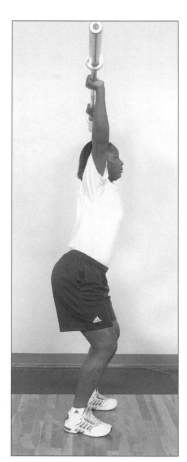

PLYOMETRICS

So how do plyometrics work? Plyometric exercises stimulate nerves and muscles to create greater amounts of explosive force. During a plyometric exercise, we place muscles on a rapid prestretch to elicit a more forceful muscle contraction. This phenomenon is called the stretch reflex. When a muscle is stretched rapidly it automatically contracts at a greater rate. Muscles, when stretched in a lengthening contraction, store energy. When athletes train using the stretch reflex mechanism, they develop explosiveness and quickness. Strength training alone cannot accomplish this result.

If we took a rubber band and stretched it, what would it do? It would snap back. Our muscles are made in the same way. Plyometric exercises work these physiological systems and increase the ability for muscles to fire more rapidly. For example, think of a volleyball player's arm in the cocking phase just before the spike. The muscles of the chest and shoulder are put on a rapid stretch just before the forward swing of the arm. The gather of a basketball player just before she elevates into her jump shot is another example. In this example, the athlete's quadriceps are placed on a rapid stretch immediately followed by a rapid contraction.

Plyometric Safety

Keep several things in mind before adding plyometric drills to your routine. This will ensure that you execute the drills safely.

Surface. Perform drills on a flat, smooth surface that has some give, but is not soft. For example, soft wooden courts, rubberized track surfaces, and grass fields that are even are good choices. Avoid hard surfaces such as concrete or tarten (hard rubber) courts.

Footwear. Wear shoes with cushioned soles that provide lateral support. Wear a basketball or cross-training shoe for multidirectional drills. Running shoes are appropriate for linear drills such as bounding.

Supervision. High school or younger athletes should be closely supervised, and they need constant feedback. Partners or coaches should provide spotting. Plyometrics should not be used with prepubescent athletes; however, you can incorporate low-intensity drills such as hops and skips into team training time for prepubescent athletes.Remember, this book lists only some of the drills used by athletes. Others such as hopscotch incorporate the stretch reflex and are considered low-intensity plyometrics appropriate for young female athletes. Athletes who exhibit base strength or who have been on a strength training program can initiate a low-intensity program and progress as they master skills.

Intensity. Plyometric drills have been developed across a range of intensities. Athletes should perform low-level exercises first and progress as their strength increases, making sure they maintain proper technique as the exercises become more intense.

History. An athlete with a history of injuries should consult her athletic trainer and physician before starting a plyometric program. She also needs close supervision.

Strength base. All athletes performing plyometric drills must have an adequate strength base. A coach can use several methods to determine if an advanced athlete (high school or above) is ready to start plyometrics. Some coaches say that an athlete should be able to parallel squat one and one-half times her body weight before initiating a plyometrics program. This rule is sound, but we believe that an athlete can begin plyometric training when she exhibits proper technique in the core lifts. These lifts include front and back squats, Romanian deadlifts, and hang cleans with a bar. When the athlete exhibits proper balance and body position, she is ready to start a low- to moderate-intensity training regimen. Plyometric drills should be used as part of the strength training regimen, but not act as a substitute.

Warm-up. Perform the dynamic warm-up provided in chapter 8 before starting plyometric drills.

Progression. Perform plyometric drills as a workout or in conjunction with a strength or power routine. Perform these exercises early in the workout. Plyometric training stimulates muscles through neural pathways; therefore, muscles and nerves must be fresh to reap the most benefit.

Equipment. Make sure all equipment is safe—that boxes are stable, medicine balls have grip, and barriers are soft and forgiving.

Plyometric Drills

The drills that follow can be incorporated into your existing training program or used with the preseason speed and agility training program detailed on page 118. The drills presented are classified as low-intensity, moderate-intensity, or high-intensity.

We defined the parameters for performing plyometrics in the beginning of this chapter. We also discussed safety issues. Another important training aspect for athletes and coaches to recognize, perhaps the most important, is intensity.

Low- to moderate-intensity drills are performed in-season and are used for maintenance. They stimulate the nervous system and promote balance and fitness. High-intensity drills are best performed during the later cycles in the off-season and throughout the preseason to develop speed power, balance, and timing. Full rest must follow high-intensity exercise to allow muscles to recover and regain full physiological capacity. Athletes should give themselves 72 hours between high-intensity workouts.

You can perform plyometric drills year-round, but choose the type of drill, level of intensity, and volume according to the season. Table 7.1 provides a simple guideline for working plyometrics into a seasonal training plan.

Table 7.1 Periodization Scheme for Plyometrics Program

Season	Duration (weeks)	Intensity	Volume (contacts/session)	Sessions (per week)	Recovery between sessions (hours)
General	12	Low	80-120	1 or 2	72
Off-season	12-24	Moderate to High	60-100	2 or 3	48-72
Preseason	4-6	High	50-80	2 or 3	48-72
In-season	12-24	Moderate to High	40-80	1 or 2	72

LOW-INTENSITY DRILLS

FRONT-TO-BACK BARRIER HOPS

This drill trains reaction off the ground and body positioning, skills needed when stopping and starting. Coaches can use this beginner drill to teach short ground time (the amount of time the feet spend on the ground).

1. Place a six- to eight-inch-high (15- to 20-centimeter-high) foam barrier on the ground in front of you.

2. Start by jumping over the barrier and landing on the balls of the feet with ankles stable. Keep the hands and arms close to the body and use a quick, explosive arm action to lead each jump.

3. Rapidly rebound off the surface, jumping back to the start position.

4. Perform two sets of 15 contacts.

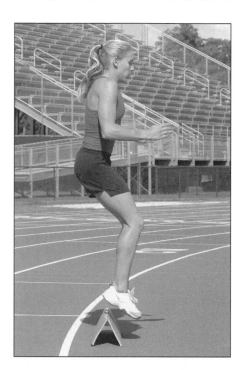

SIDE-TO-SIDE BARRIER HOPS

This drill is especially effective for developing explosive cuts off the outside foot. Soccer, field hockey, and basketball players should use this drill.

1. Place a six- to eight-inch-high (15- to 20-centimeter-high) foam barrier on the ground to your right.

2. Start by jumping over the barrier to the right.

3. As soon as the balls of the feet touch the ground, jump over the barrier to the left.

4. Perform the drill on the balls of the feet and with aggressive arm action.

5. Perform two sets of 15 contacts.

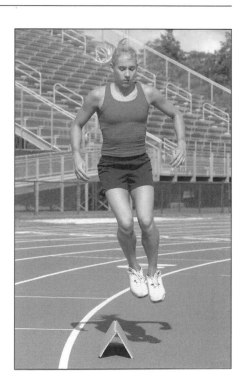

BOX RUN SHUFFLE

This drill develops quickness and stability in rapid foot movements. You need a sturdy wooden or metal box that is six to eight inches (15 to 20 centimeters) high and preferably two feet (about a half-meter) × two feet wide.

1. Start by facing the box with one foot on the box and the other on the ground.
2. Keep the arms in front in a ready position to help maintain balance.
3. Quickly move the foot that was on the box to the ground and the foot that was on the ground to the box.
4. Rebound off the ground like you are running in place.
5. Maintain balance and a good athletic position. Move the arms and legs in opposition.
6. Perform two sets of 10 contacts.

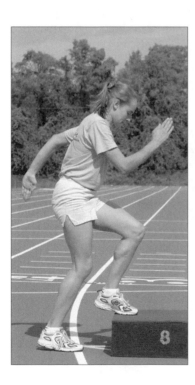 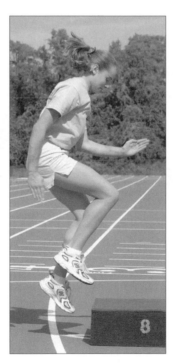 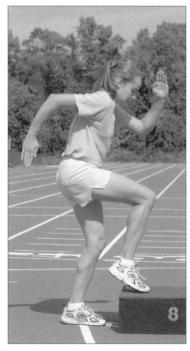

QUICK-RESPONSE JUMP

This drill shortens an athlete's ground time during running and jumping. It also teaches athletes to maintain balance and center of gravity. An added benefit is that athletes develop proper arm and leg coordination as the arms gather and lead the legs.

1. Stand facing a six-inch-high (15-centimeter-high) box. Start by jumping off the ground with both feet onto the box and then back down. Stay on the balls of the feet and use the arms to initiate the upward movement.

2. Perform these jumps in rapid succession. Stay on the balls of the feet with stable ankles.

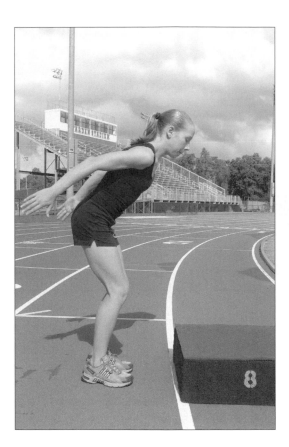 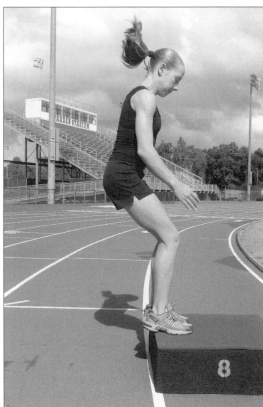

MODERATE-INTENSITY DRILLS

TUCK JUMP

The tuck jump works on jumping and quickness off the ground.

1. Start from a standing position on a smooth, pliable surface.
2. Explode straight up off the ground, initiating the jump with the arms.
3. After leaving the ground, drive the knees up so that the upper thighs are parallel to the jump surface and the arms are straight out at shoulder height.
4. When the body starts its downward movement, aggressively thrust the legs toward the ground and contact the surface. Rebound off the surface immediately and repeat the jump.
5. Perform two sets of six to eight repetitions.

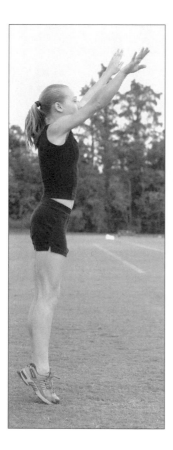
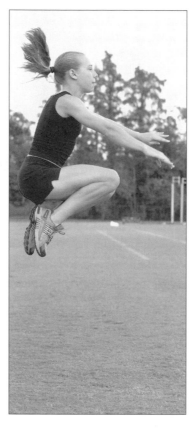
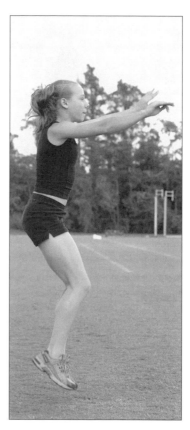

SPLIT JUMP

Split jumps develop power in the gluteals, hamstrings, and hip flexors. They help develop balance as well.

1. Stand with the legs in a stride position (left leg forward, right leg back).
2. Explode upward off the ground, jumping as high as possible.
3. Scissor the legs in the air and land with the opposite leg forward.
4. Perform 10 ground contacts (five per leg) and repeat for two sets

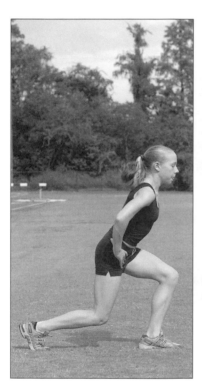 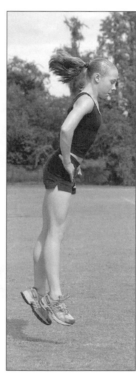 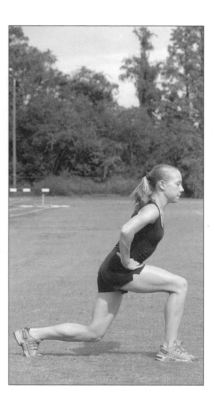

BOX JUMP FOR HEIGHT

Box jumps for height help develop quickness off the ground and teach proper body landing position. The focus of this drill is the jump up onto the box. Make sure you use a stable sturdy box with a cushioned top. Box heights vary from 14 to 24 inches (30 to 60 centimeters) based on the ability of each athlete.

1. Start by facing a box about 16 inches (about 40 centimeters) high.
2. Explode up off the ground getting as high as you can so that you must come down on the box to land. Use an aggressive upward swing of the arms to lead the jump.
3. Land flat-footed on the box in a good athletic position with knees bent slightly, chest over the knees, and feet shoulder-width apart.
4. Perform three jumps for three different box heights for nine total contacts. Increase the box heights when you can complete the highest box comfortably.

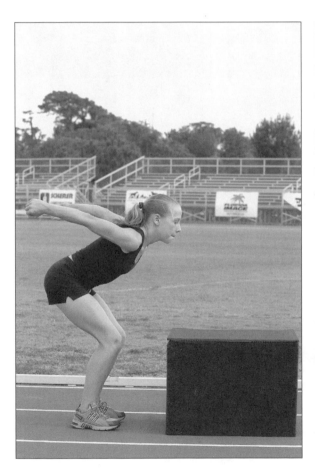 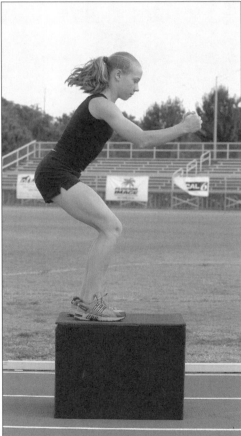

SQUAT JUMP

Basketball players benefit from this exercise when rebounding, and swimmers feel its effects when exploding off the blocks or pushing off the wall during turns. It is also good for goal-keepers in soccer.

1. Start in a half-squat position (with the knees at 90 degrees and hips at 45 degrees). Place the hands behind the head.
2. Explode up off the ground.
3. Jump vertically, driving the body to a fully extended position.
4. Land in the same position as the takeoff with feet shoulder-width apart.
5. Perform two sets of 10 jumps.

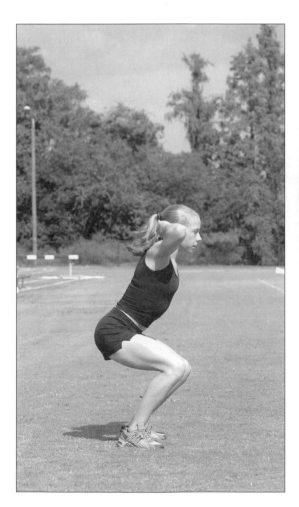
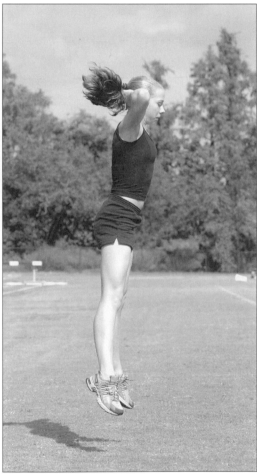

LATERAL BOX SHUFFLE

This drill develops lateral explosiveness and agility. It teaches proper body mechanics during changes in direction. It is especially good for basketball and volleyball players.

1. Start by standing next to a six- to eight-inch-high (15- to 20-centimeter-high) sturdy box with one foot on the box and the other foot on the ground.
2. Begin with the arms in a ready position.
3. Explode off the inside foot (the foot on the box), and drive off the box, staying as low to the box as possible. Move across the box so that the other foot lands on the box and the original working foot lands on the floor. Stay balanced by maintaining a good athletic position.
4. Rebound off the floor and change direction from the right to the left.
5. Perform 8 to 10 repetitions and complete two sets.

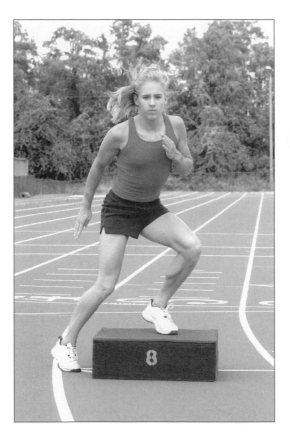 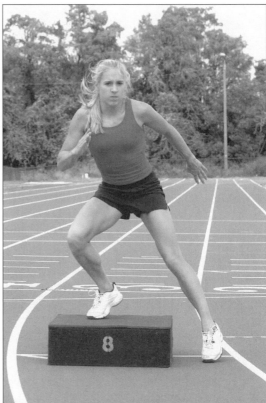

HIGH-INTENSITY DRILLS

Bounding is one of the best high-intensity plyometric drills. It was detailed in chapter 6 (page 105) because it develops stride length and efficient running form. Bounding is an overexaggeration of the running stride that helps increase an athlete's stride length and overall speed. It takes a lot of muscle strength to stabilize the body during bounding drills.

SINGLE-LEG BOUNDING

Bounding improves an athlete's overall athleticism and power in all sports, but it should become a training mainstay for sprinters, jumpers, or athletes in any sport requiring sprinting and jumping.

1. Start with several approach steps to gain momentum.
2. Take off on one leg, driving off the ground, and leading with the arms.
3. The arms work together by gathering in a circular motion. As they drive forward, the working leg follows.
4. Elevate the takeoff leg to parallel, and finish by contacting the ground on the ball of the same foot with the toes at or slightly behind the knee.
5. Perform two sets of four to six bounds on each leg.

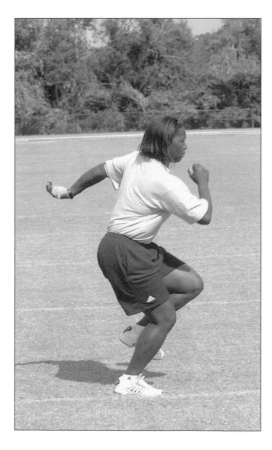
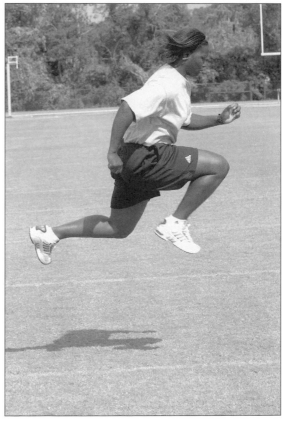

CYCLE HOPS

When running, the legs move in a a circular motion. Cycle hops train this specific technique. To perform this drill correctly the athlete must elevate her knee parallel to the ground and pull the heel to the gluteal muscles. This creates the circular motion needed for explosive running. The downward movement of the foot creates a "pawing" of the ground and must occur rapidly. This drill is one of the most difficult and requires strength, speed, balance, and rhythm. Include this drill in the training of any athlete who must run fast, but only if she is ready to perform it. Cycle hops are an advanced version of the single-leg bound. They are performed at a much faster speed, and the primary goal is not to cover ground but to complete the circular motion of the leg as explosively as possible.

1. Start the movement in a standing position. Take one approach step and drive the working leg upward, bringing the thigh parallel to the ground and the heel straight up to the gluteal muscles.

2. Land on the ball of the same foot. Begin by doing one cycle hop at a time and work up to multiple repetition sets so that the drill is always performed rapidly. Move arms in opposition to the legs.

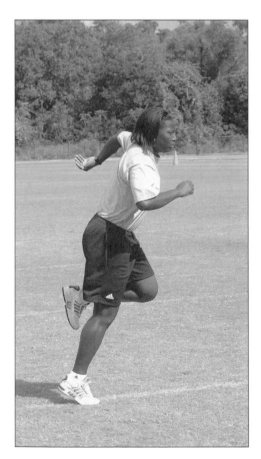 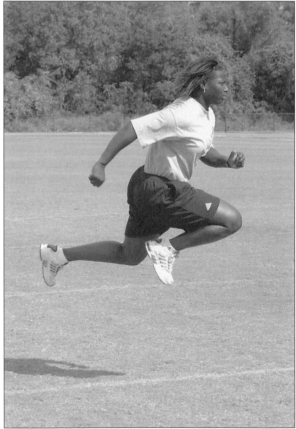

While most of the plyometric drills described in this chapter work the lower body, other total-body exercises train explosiveness in upper-body movements. Some of the best exercises for the upper body (in addition to the Olympic lifts discussed at the beginning of this chapter) are the medicine ball chest passes and overhead throws (see chapter 5).

The same principles apply to upper-body plyometrics as apply to lower-body drills. The catch or recovery phase is rapid. Place the working muscles on a rapid stretch, and elicit a rapid and forceful contraction of the muscle creating the opposite movement. When performing these drills, be sure to keep your back flat and abdominal muscles tight, and maintain a good working base with your legs. Upper-body plyometrics help increase the velocity of throwing, striking, twisting, passing, and shooting, and they are particularly good for basketball and volleyball players.

When you perform upper-body plyometrics using medicine balls, remember not to use too much weight. These drills should focus on speed and technique. Because the weight used is not as important, begin these exercises using a weight light enough to allow you to maintain proper technique.

Before performing the plyometric program outlined in table 7.2, review and become familiar with all the safety rules associated with plyometric training (see page 123). Make sure you have been performing a minimum of six weeks of strength training and have a good strength base before starting any plyometric work. Work to execute all drills with proper technique first, and consider increasing the intensity only after you have achieved proper technique.

The program provided is a 12-week periodized off-season plyometric program. It should be initiated during the second half of your off-season training, leading into your preseason work. Notice that the intensities are low at the beginning and high at the end of the program. Stay with the given progression; do not try to add more exercises beyond what you see here. Perform the program on alternate days of strength training, twice each week, and always start with a proper warm-up (see chapter 8).

Table 7.2 12-Week Off-Season Plyometric Program

Week*	1	2	3	4	5
Level of intensity	Low	Low	Low to moderate	Moderate	Moderate
Exercise	Sets × reps				
Barrier hops (front/back)	2 × 15	2 × 15	2 × 10	–	–
Barrier hops (side/side)	2 × 15	2 × 15	2 × 10	2 × 10	2 × 10
Lateral box shuffle	2 × 15	2 × 20	2 × 10	2 × 10	2 × 10
Quick-response jump	2 × 15	2 × 15	2 × 10	–	–
Tuck jump	–	–	2 × 8	2 × 8	3 × 8
Split jump (each leg)	–	–	2 × 8	2 × 10	3 × 8
Squat jump	–	–	2 × 8	2 × 10	3 × 8
Box jump for height **	–	–	–	1 × 4 @ 14, 16, and 18"	1 × 4 @ 14, 16, 18, and 20"
Bounding (diagonal skate)	–	–	–	–	3 × 10
Bounding	–	–	–	–	–
Single-leg bounding	–	–	–	–	–
Cycle hops	–	–	–	–	–
Medicine ball: chest pass***	2 × 15	2 × 15	2 × 15	2 × 20	2 × 20
Medicine ball: overhead throw***	2 × 15	2 × 15	2 × 15	2 × 20	2 × 20
Medicine ball: twist pass***	2 × 15	2 × 15	2 × 15	2 × 20	2 × 20

* Perform two workouts each week.

** Box jump for height: Heights are only a recommendation. Set your box height where it is comfortable and where you can maintain proper technique.

*** Increase the weight of the medicine balls after week 8.

1 inch = 2.54 centimeters

6	7	8	9	10	11	12
Moderate	Moderate	Moderate to advanced	Moderate to advanced	Moderate to advanced	Advanced	Advanced
-	-	-	-	-	-	-
-	-	-	-	-	-	-
-	-	-	-	-	2 × 8	2 × 8
-	-	-	-	-	-	-
3 × 8	2 × 8	3 × 8	3 × 8	3 × 8	3 × 8	3 × 8
3 × 8	2 × 8	3 × 8	-	-	-	-
3 × 8	2 × 8	-	-	-	-	-
1 × 4 @ 16, 18, 20, and 22"	1 × 4 @ 16, 18, 20, and 22"	1 × 5 @ 18, 20, and 22"	1 × 5 @ 18, 20, and 22"	1 × 5 @ 18, 20, 22, and 24"	-	-
3 × 10	2 × 10	3 × 10	3 × 10	3 × 10	3 × 8 weighted	3 × 8 weighted
-	3 × 4	3 × 4	3 × 4	3 × 5	3 × 5	3 × 5
-	-	-	3 × 4	3 × 5	-	-
-	-	-	-	-	2 × 5	2 × 5
2 × 20	2 × 20	2 × 20	2 × 15	2 × 15	2 × 15	2 × 20
2 × 20	2 × 20	2 × 20	2 × 15	2 × 15	2 × 15	2 × 20
2 × 20	2 × 20	2 × 20	2 × 15	2 × 15	2 × 15	2 × 20

Part IV
Training for Performance

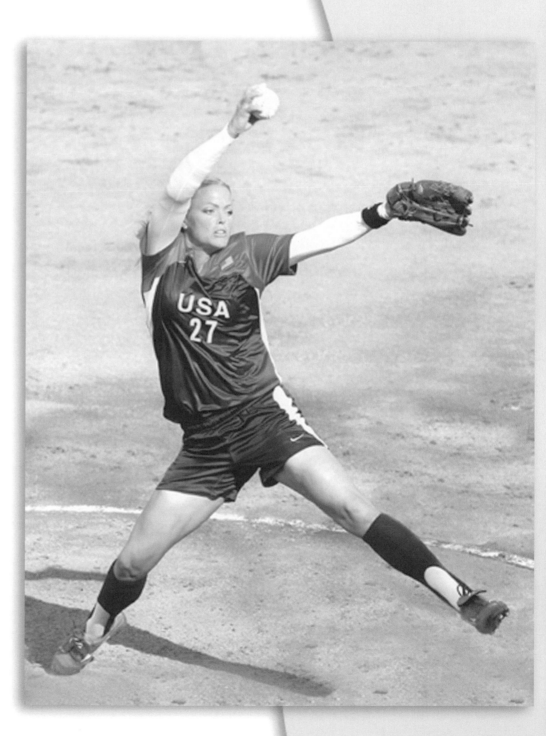

8

Preparing for High-Intensity Training

Over the past 10 years the way athletes warm up for training has changed significantly. In the past most teams began practice by running a lap or two around the field or court followed by 10 minutes of static stretching. Most of the warm-up seemed to be for the mouth.

Social time at the beginning of practice is fine, but not at the expense of a proper warm-up. And although static stretching is valuable for increasing flexibility and has a place *within* a proper warm-up, its primary merits occur when it is done at the end of a training session, during the cool-down.

In our experience working with athletes from the youth to elite levels, the first 15 minutes of a training session prepare the athlete's body for the physical stress of a practice session. This is the objective of a proper warm-up—to increase the body's core temperature by performing dynamic drills. Static stretching alone does little to prepare muscles for intense exercise. Recent research suggests that long bouts of static stretching before exercise may actually make muscles lethargic. A dynamic warm-up on the other hand serves two primary purposes:

1. Improve performance.
   - Dynamic movements increase core temperature. Dynamic movements increase the flow of blood and oxygen to working muscles and stimulate nerve firing. These actions prepare the body for competition.
   - The best warm-up activities also develop skills. Many coaches and athletes struggle to find adequate warm-up time. Some coaches exclude a proper warm-up, preferring to use this time for skills training. Performing specific skill training at submaximal levels as a warm-up accomplishes two tasks— warming up the muscles and developing sport-specific skills.
   - A dynamic warm-up reduces muscle tension. Muscles that are warm and loose are more efficient. Warmed-up muscles contract more effectively and are able to move through a full range of motion with less risk of injury.

- A dynamic warm-up promotes psychological readiness. Teams tend to start workouts with static stretching. Oftentimes these stretching sessions turn into social periods. Some coaches promote this social time and that's fine, but many teams lose focus during this period. Dynamic work is a perfect mental and physical transition for athletes as they move from low- to higher- intensity training.

2. Decrease risk of injuries. As an athlete, you are always at risk for injury, but proper preparation will help you avoid it. Increasing blood flow and O_2, decreasing muscle tension (increasing ROM), and being more mentally focused all contribute to staying injury free.

   - A dynamic warm-up may decrease the incidence of muscle and ligament strains and sprains.

   - A dynamic warm-up reduces the risk of overuse injuries. Overuse injuries typically occur with repetitive bouts of exercise or trauma to a specific area of the body. For example, patellar tendinitis occurs in athletes who jump repetitively over time. Repetitive trauma causes microtears in the soft tissue and a build-up of chemical waste products around the area. Warm-up, however, tends to ready these high-stress areas by bringing fresh blood and oxygen to the area and removing waste products built up in the muscles. Skipping the warm-up session allows waste to build until the joint eventually breaks down.

   - Although it has not yet been proven scientifically that warming up reduces muscle soreness, we know from our years as athletes and coaches that this seems to be the case. We hear athletes commenting every day about how the warm-up made them feel better. The benefits of dynamic warm-up that appear to decrease the risk of overuse injuries also appear to play a major role in triggering this response of feeling better.

Some coaches or athletes may complain, "But, I don't have 15 minutes to waste in the beginning of practice on warming up." Our answer to that is this: The warm-up in this chapter may just be the most important 15 minutes you spend during a practice session. Beverly Buckley, head coach of women's tennis at Rollins College agrees: "The dynamic warm-up has become an integral part of my team's program and has been effective in preparing the athletes both mentally and physically for practice and game situations."

POWER WARM-UP

The power warm-up we have devised can be broken into four parts done over 15 minutes at the start of any practice, game, or competition.

General warm-up is usually the earliest portion of the warm-up process. During this stage the athlete elevates her core temperature by performing physical activities such as light jogging, easy rope jumping, or calisthenic-type exercises.

Static stretching, also called hold stretching, is used primarily to increase muscle flexibility and range of motion around a joint. Short static stretches are appropriate for part of the warm-up, but are most effective during the cool-down.

Dynamic stretching is moving a muscle through a range of motion to help increase the core temperature of that muscle and to stimulate neural function. Dynamic programs increase the athlete's preparedness and provide a perfect transition from the resting state to full competition activity.

Speed-and-movement drills are designed to increase muscle temperature while helping the athlete develop specific skill techniques. Drills for speed and agility are used for running sports. These drills also help athletes develop balance and timing. Dynamic movements like running or fast-feet drills are most effective when muscles and nerves are fresh, but properly warm and limber. Athletes should always work on motor skill drills early in practice, after a general warm-up, to maximize motor learning.

As with all training, determining the order of exercises is crucial. Athletes should perform complex movements involving large muscle groups first, followed by single joint exercises. We recommend this for several reasons. If an athlete exhausts the triceps by doing a triceps-only exercise first, then performing the bench press, which includes the triceps as well as other chest muscles, becomes more difficult. The idea is to work the muscles from the inside (center of the body) outward. The large muscle groups are most important because they provide the foundation for movement and strength for the extremities. Another reason to work the complex movements first is that these optimally train the nervous system. We want to work movements that incorporate the kinetic chain and multijoint movements. Work the nervous system when it is fresh so that motor learning is optimized.

Warming up the human body is like firing up an old Apollo rocket. Those rockets worked through several stages before they were ready for liftoff. The largest stages were the most powerful and always fired first, followed by the smaller rockets that fine-tuned the movements. The smallest stages would not have been able to perform without the more powerful stages leading the way. Let's look at the example of a world-class female shot putter. Her legs, the largest stage, create the initial explosion. From there power is transferred through the hips to the torso, shoulders, arms, and finally the index finger, the smallest stage. In this scenario the follow-through of the shot put at the wrist and fingers is no less important than the initial drive off the leg, but its efficiency is totally dependent on the power generated at the largest stage, the legs.

Table 8.1 summarizes the power warm-up. The specific ideas that follow will help each athlete optimize her potential for performance in her sport.

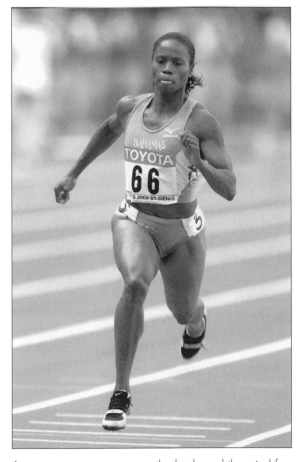

A proper warm-up prepares the body and the mind for intense exercise or competition.

Table 8.1 Power Warm-Up

Component	Exercise	Details and duration
General warm-up (3 min)	Jog	Multidirectional
Static stretching (5 min)	Hamstring stretch: straddle position Side lunge Iliotibial band stretch Forward lunge Groin stretch Quadriceps stretch Calf stretch Partner chest stretch* Latissimus dorsi stretch* Prayer and seal stretches*	Hold each for 15 seconds. Be sure to stretch left and right sides.
Dynamic range-of-motion drills (3 min)	Side leg swing Forward–backward leg swing Knee–ankle swivel Trunk twist* Small arm circles* Full-ROM arm circles*	Perform 1 set of 15 for each side.
Dynamic speed-and-movement drills (5 min)	High-knee skip Heel kick Straight-leg toe touch Carioca Backward stride Fast-feet: backpedal Fast-feet: forward Fast-feet: sideways Fast-feet: forward, backward, forward	Perform 2 sets of 15 yards for each.

* These exercises are optional.

General Warm-Up

Start any warm-up with three to five minutes of general submaximal exercises. This increases the body's core temperature. The general warm-up varies based on your sport or whether you are an individual or part of a team. Multidirectional jogging, stationary bicycling, jumping rope, or general sport drills like shooting jump shots are examples of general warm-up activities.

Static Stretching

Perform a series of static stretches from a standing position for five minutes. This will act as a transition into more aggressive dynamic movements. It is also a good time for coaches to bring the team together at the beginning of practice. We recommend standing stretches rather than seated because they prevent athletes from losing concentration and becoming lethargic. Throughout the following routine, move from one static stretch to the next without hesitation. Perform only one set of stretches, holding each for 15 seconds.

LOWER-BODY STRETCHES

These are appropriate before any sport.

HAMSTRING STRETCH: STRADDLE POSITION

This stretch focuses on the hamstrings, gluteals, and muscles of the low back.

1. Stand in a straddle position with feet three to five feet apart.
2. Keep the knees slightly bent and toes pointed outward at a 45-degree angle.
3. Slowly bend from the waist, bringing the chest toward one knee and keeping the back flat.
4. Stretch to one side until you feel tension in the hamstrings and hold.
5. Perform this stretch toward the opposite knee and the center.

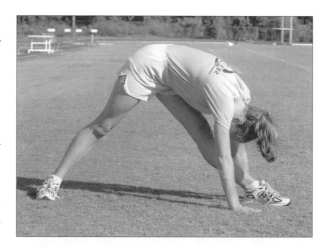

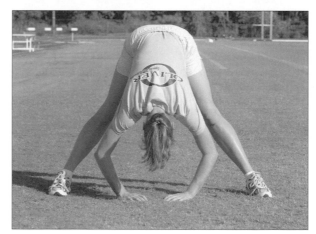

SIDE LUNGE STRETCH

This exercise stretches the thigh adductors (groin) and hamstrings.

1. Start in a standing straddle position.
2. Facing forward, slowly lunge to the left.
3. Keep the back flat and the toes pointed forward. The knee of the lunging leg should fall directly over the toes, not past them.
4. Repeat on the other side.

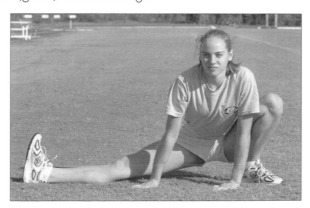

ILIOTIBIAL BAND STRETCH

This stretch focuses on the tensor fasciae latae, gluteals, iliotibial band, and muscles of the low back.

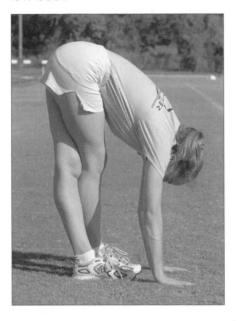

1. Start in a standing position.
2. Cross the right leg over the left.
3. Keep the knees slightly bent.
4. Slowly bend at the waist toward the right, reaching down with the right hand toward the ankle of the back foot.
5. Repeat the stretch with the left leg crossed over the right.

FORWARD LUNGE STRETCH

This stretch works the hip flexors and gluteals.

1. Start with an upright posture, abs tight, and shoulders back, arms at your side.
2. Take a large step forward with the right leg (lead leg) and plant the right foot flat on the floor. Allow the left knee to bend slightly.
3. Drop your body down to bend the right knee slightly beyond a 90-degree angle. Make sure that the front knee is directly over the front foot.

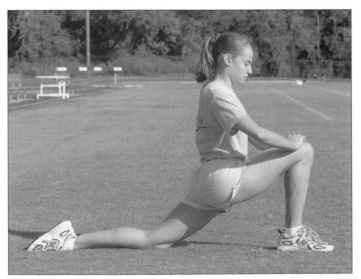

4. Slowly shift your weight forward while pressing the hip of the back leg toward the ground.
5. Return to the starting position and repeat the exercise with the opposite leg.

GROIN STRETCH

This stretch focuses on the adductor muscle group (groin).

1. From a standing position slowly drop into a full squat position so that the toes are pointed out at 45 degrees.
2. With a flat back, push the knees outward with the elbows.

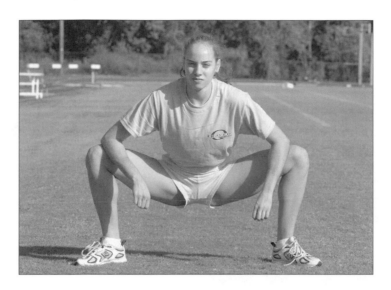

QUADRICEPS STRETCH

This stretch focuses on the quadriceps muscle group and the hip flexors.

1. From a standing position, balance yourself by holding onto a wall, chair, other stationary object, or partner.
2. Grasp the right foot and pull the heel toward the gluteal muscles.
3. Push the right hip forward to get a better hip flexor stretch.
4. Switch legs and repeat.

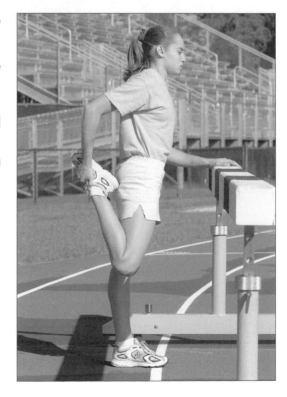

CALF STRETCH

This stretch focuses on the gastrocnemius and soleus muscles.

1. In a standing position with the right leg lunging forward, support yourself by placing the hands in front of you on a wall or other stationary object.
2. Press the heel of the back leg toward the floor while keeping the leg straight (to stretch just the gastrocnemius).
3. Switch sides and repeat.
4. Bend the knee of the back leg to stretch the soleus muscle.

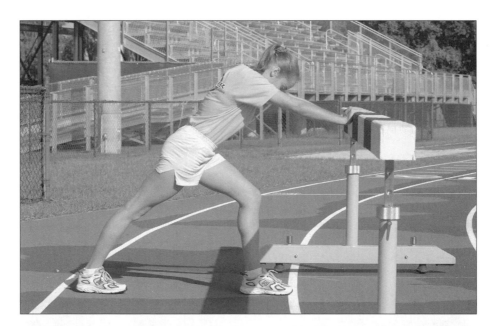

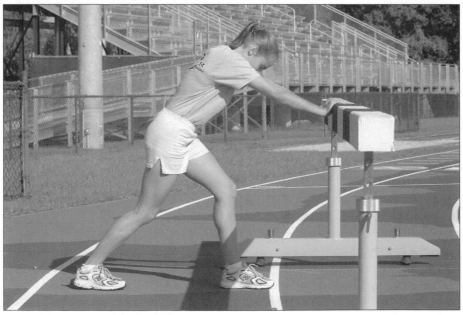

UPPER-BODY STRETCHES

The following upper-body stretches are appropriate for all sports for total-body flexibility, but are especially important for throwing sports and swimming.

PARTNER CHEST STRETCH

This stretch focuses on the biceps, anterior deltoid, and pectoralis muscles.

1. While standing, have a partner grasp your arms at the wrists behind your body.
2. The partner slowly raises the arms upward until you feel a stretch at the front deltoids and outside chest.

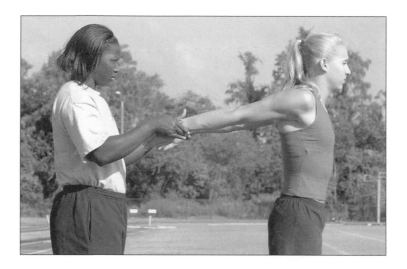

LATISSIMUS DORSI STRETCH

This stretch focuses on the latissimus dorsi and triceps.

1. In a standing position, bend the right arm behind you and touch the middle of the back.
2. Keep the upper arm perpendicular to the ground with the elbow pointing up.
3. Switch sides and repeat.

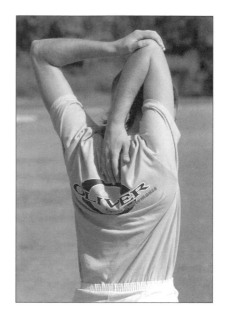

PRAYER AND SEAL STRETCHES

This set of stretches focuses on the forearm flexors (prayer) and the forearm extensors (seal).

1. While standing, place the hands together in front of the chest with the palms touching and fingertips pointing upward.
2. With the hands together, press the palms together and downward toward your navel until you feel a stretch.
3. For the seal stretch, touch the back sides of your hands together in front of your chest with the fingertips pointing downward.
4. Press the back sides together as you lower the hands downward toward your navel.

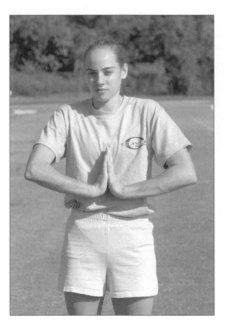 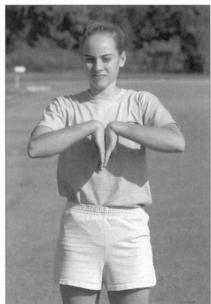

DYNAMIC RANGE-OF-MOTION DRILLS

The next part of the warm-up consists of dynamic range-of-motion drills. These exercises are more aggressive and are performed through a greater range of motion to prepare the nervous system for more vigorous activity. These drills not only increase muscle temperature, but they also stimulate neural firing of muscle groups. The following drills include movements that work the lower and upper body.

SIDE LEG SWING

This drill works the abductors and adductors.

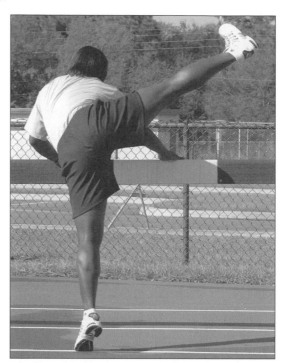

1. With hands on a wall or holding onto a rail, position your body so that you are two to three feet from the wall or rail.

2. Starting on the right side, swing the right leg from side to side like a pendulum. As the leg moves to the inside, point the toes in. As the leg moves outward, point the toes out.

3. While swinging the leg from side to side, make sure to swivel the hips with the movement.

4. Kick the leg up to a point where you feel a stretch in the adductors (groin).

5. Switch legs and repeat for both sides.

6. Perform 10 to 15 swings for each leg.

FORWARD–BACKWARD LEG SWING

This drill works the hamstrings and hip flexors.

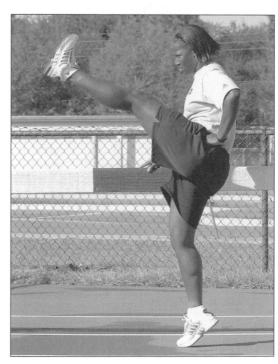

1. With the right shoulder facing the wall, place the right hand on the wall to support yourself.

2. Start by swinging the left leg forward until you feel a stretch in the hamstring and then backward until you feel a stretch in the hip flexor (front hip).

3. Maintain an upright posture through the movement.

4. Switch legs (turn around and face the other way) and repeat.

5. Perform 10 to 15 repetitions.

KNEE–ANKLE SWIVEL

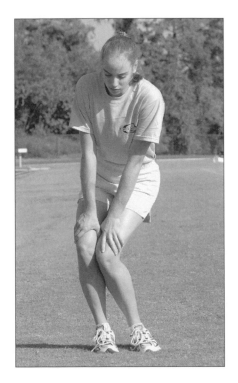

This drill works all the lower-extremity muscles around the hip, knee, and ankle joints.

1. Start in a standing position with the legs together and knees bent slightly.
2. Place the hands on the knees.
3. Move the knees in a circular motion while keeping the feet flat on the ground.
4. Perform this drill circling to the right and then to the left.
5. Perform 10 to 15 circles in each direction.

SMALL ARM CIRCLES

This drill works the muscles of the rotator cuff and trapezius.

1. Start in a standing position with the knees bent slightly and arms straight out at the sides.
2. Rotate the arms in a circular motion forward and then back.
3. Start with slow movements and progress to rapid circles.
4. Perform 15 circles each direction with each arm.

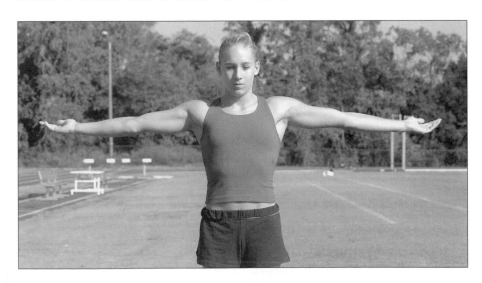

FULL-ROM ARM CIRCLES

This drill works the muscles of the rotator cuff and trapezius through a full range of motion.

1. From a standing position with the knees slightly bent, hold the arms out in front parallel to the floor, then rotate the arms backward making full circles.
2. Perform this drill with the arms rotating in the same direction.
3. Perform this drill with the arms rotating in opposite directions—one arm rotating forward while the other arm rotates backward.
4. Perform 15 circles in each direction with each arm.

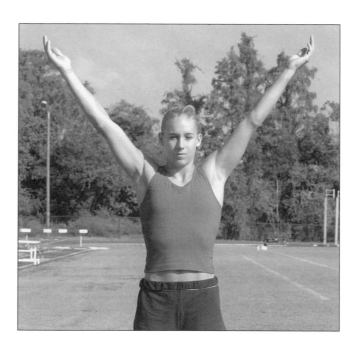

TRUNK TWIST

This drill works the obliques (side abdominals), pectoralis, and low back muscles.

1. Place a broomstick, golf club, lacrosse stick, or similarly sized straight stick behind the neck and grasp the ends of the stick with the hands. The stick should be long enough to grasp with the hands.
2. While maintaining an upright posture with slightly bent knees, slowly rotate from left to right, then from right to left, obtaining the fullest range of motion possible.
3. Increase the speed throughout the range of motion as you feel comfortable.
4. Perform 10 to 15 rotations

DYNAMIC SPEED AND MOVEMENT DRILLS

The dynamic speed and movement drills presented here complete the warm-up. These drills develop running technique and include more sport-specific skills. For example, the fast-feet drills develop muscle memory, rhythm, and timing and act as a great transition from the warm-up to full-speed practice.

BACKWARD STRIDE

This drill works the gluteal muscles and the hamstrings.

1. From an athletic position start the movement by striding backward.
2. Push off the ground aggressively with the front leg while raising the opposite leg heel-up toward the gluteals and then straight back.
3. Use aggressive arm action with the arms working in opposition to the legs (right arm forward, left leg back).
4. Cover 15 to 20 yards or meters and repeat.

FAST-FEET: FORWARD

This drill works the quadriceps, calves, and anterior tibialis muscles.

1. Start from an athletic position with the feet about 12 inches (30 centimeters) apart and staggered.
2. On the first go signal move the feet as rapidly as possible with rhythmic ground contacts while moving forward.
3. Maintain a stable ankle, and perform the drill on the balls of the feet. Move the feet and arms in opposition.
4. On the second go signal (after about two to three yards or meters) plant the foot and explode into a sprint for 15 yards or meters. The planted foot should step straight down and not back from the body.
5. Perform this drill two to four times.

FAST-FEET: SIDEWAYS

This drill works the quadriceps, adductors, abductors, calves, and anterior tibialis muscles.

1. Start from an athletic position with the feet about 12 inches (30 centimeters) apart and staggered.
2. On the go signal move the feet as rapidly as possible, moving to the right or left with rhythmic ground contacts.
3. Maintain a stable ankle, and perform the drill on the balls of the feet. Move the feet and arms in opposition.
4. On the second go signal (after you have moved two to three yards or meters to the side) plant the back foot, drive off it, and turn the hips so that you can sprint forward for 15 yards or meters.
5. Perform this drill two to four times.

FAST-FEET: BACKPEDAL

This drill works the hamstrings, calves, and anterior tibialis muscles.

1. Start in an athletic position with the knees slightly bent, the back flat, the chest forward, and the hips down.
2. Aggressively backpedal with rapid foot contacts and arm action.
3. Cover 15 to 20 yards or meters and repeat.

FAST-FEET: FORWARD, BACKWARD, FORWARD

This drill works all of the muscles of the lower extremity.

1. Start from an athletic position with the feet about 12 inches (30 centimeters) apart and staggered.
2. On the first go signal move the feet as rapidly as possible with rhythmic ground contacts as you move forward.
3. Maintain a stable ankle and perform the drill on the balls of the feet. Move the feet and arms in opposition.
4. On the second go signal (after about two to three yards or meters) move the feet as rapidly as possible moving backward.
5. On the third go signal (after about two to three yards) plant the foot and explode into a sprint forward for 15 yards or meters. The planted foot should step straight down and not back from the body.
6. Perform this drill two to four times.

HIGH-KNEE SKIP

This drill works all muscles around the hip, knee, and ankle joints, especially emphasizing the hip flexors, hamstrings, and calves.

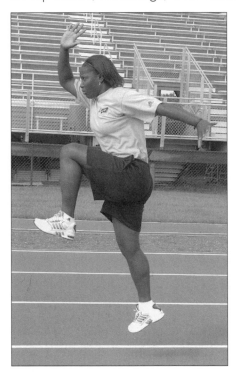

1. Perform a rhythmic skipping movement (hop step) by alternately driving the right and left knees upward.
2. Use aggressive arm movements (refer to chapter 6 for specific instructions on the arm position). Arms should swing from the shoulders.
3. Contact the ground on the ball of the foot maintaining a stable ankle position.
4. Skip 15 to 20 yards or meters and repeat.

HEEL KICK

This drill works the hamstrings, calves, and gluteal muscles.

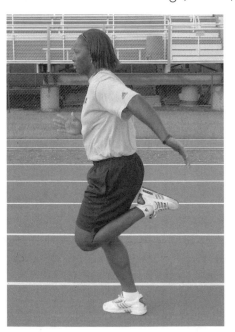

1. While moving forward, aggressively flex the knees so that the calf muscles touch the hamstrings. The thighs remain perpendicular to the ground with the ankle dorsiflexed on the upward swing of the lower leg.
2. Stay on the balls of the feet.
3. Focus on maintaining a high number of ground contacts rather than on forward speed.
4. Cover 15 to 20 yards or meters and repeat.

STRAIGHT-LEG TOE TOUCH

This drill works the hamstrings, abdominals, calves, and hip flexors.

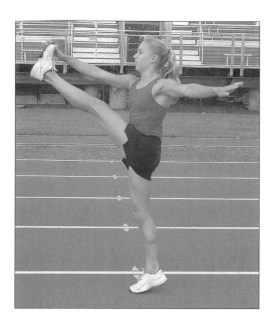

1. Hold the arms straight out from the shoulders so that they are parallel to the ground.
2. Drive the left leg upward in front, keeping the leg straight, until it touches the right hand.
3. Land on the ball of the foot, and do not let the heel touch the ground.
4. Complete the pattern with the right leg touching the left hand.
5. Cover 15 to 20 yards or meters and repeat.

CARIOCA

This drill works the abdominals (especially the obliques), low back, and hip muscles.

1. Moving laterally, swivel the hips so that the left leg crosses in front of the right.
2. Step to the side with the right leg, and complete the sequence by crossing the left leg behind the right.
3. Focus on maintaining a high number of ground contacts rather than covering ground quickly.
4. Cover 15 to 20 yards or meters leading from the left, then repeat leading from the right.

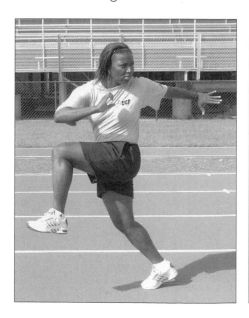
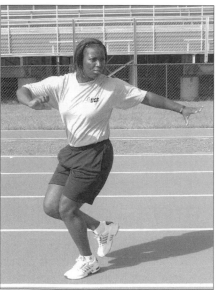
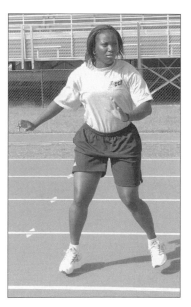

COOLING DOWN

Cooling down at the end of each workout is essential because it allows your systems to recover properly and get ready for the next practice session. This is also a great time for additional stretching. The body is most able to increase its range of motion following exercise when the muscles are hot and fatigued and more able to relax. Take 10 to 15 minutes at the end of practice to perform static stretching (see pages 152 through 158). Stretching with a partner is the most effective form of static stretching.

9

Developing Championship Workouts and Programs

Athletes often wonder how to implement a year-round training plan that helps them prepare for their specific sport. This final chapter is devoted to helping athletes lay out a systematic training schedule for building power and strength.

In this chapter we take the exercises shown in the previous chapters and detail how they can be used for a progressive strength and power training program for twelve specific sports: basketball, diving, field hockey, golf, gymnastics, lacrosse, soccer, softball, swimming, track & field (sprints and throwing events), triathlon, and volleyball. These program charts will help guide you in setting up a program that is sport-specific. Keep in mind, though, that your unique competition, training, school, and work schedules as well as other factors may require that you modify the programs slightly to fit your own needs. Always refer to proper periodization practices when making any changes to the strength and conditioning programs outlined here. Refer back to chapter 1 for guidelines on setting up all your seasons of training. Always perform proper *technique* first and then increase your intensity (speed or weight).

The program charts are broken down into three phases (as discussed in chapter 1): the off-season, preseason, and in-season. In addition several of the sports have the phases broken into training blocks—three off-season blocks, two preseason blocks and one in-season block. As with the progression of phases, these training blocks are designed to progressively prepare the athlete for more intense and sport-specific physical preparation. The off-season phase may be the most important training phase because it develops a strong base for the programs that follow. A solid off-season phase of training helps prevent injury, increase tolerance for intense exercise, develop neural patterns for explosive exercise, and increase muscle size and strength. The preseason phase starts preparing the athlete for high-intensity exercise. The exercises become more sport-specific. This phase really sets the stage for the in-season training phase, which is designed to maintain strength, power, and muscular fitness. Therefore, the preseason phase determines what level the athlete will maintain during her competitive season. Athletes should focus and work hard during all phases of training.

Any effective training program includes several specific variables. These include the type of exercise, how many sets and repetitions you do, how much rest you take between sets, and the order in which exercises are done. In each program we've set up these variables precisely; they are synchronized to produce specific results in each training session, training week, and training phase. Each exercise in each table includes the page number on which you will find the description of how to execute that exercise.

Before we get to the sport-specific programs though, we provide several tables that you will use in many of the sport-specific programs: a general abdominal and core program (table 9.1), a medicine ball and advanced core program (table 9.2), and a speed movement drills program (table 9.3). Each of these programs can also be used as a stand-alone workout.

Remember to perform a proper warm-up before any of the workouts provided here. Refer back to chapter 8 to review the components of a proper warm-up as well as some suggestions for dynamic movement drills to help prepare the muscles for high-intensity training.

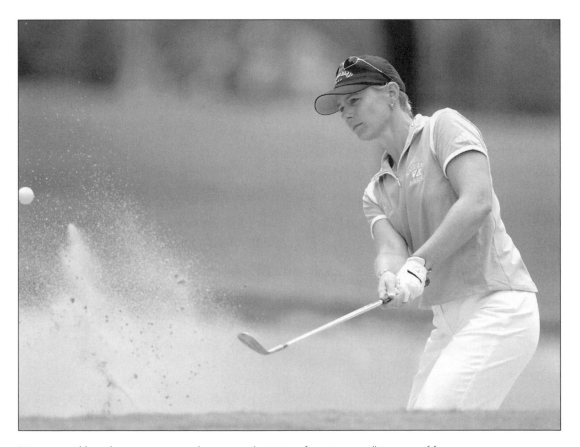

Many top athletes have incorporated year-round training, focusing on all aspects of fitness.

Table 9.1   Abdominal and Core Program A (General)

Week	1	2	3	4	5	6	7	8
Abdominal curl	3 × 20	3 × 20	3 × 25	3 × 25	3 × 30	3 × 30	3 × 35	3 × 35
Bench obliques	1 × 20	1 × 20	1 × 25	1 × 25	1 × 30	1 × 30	1 × 35	1 × 35
Reverse crunch	1 × 20	1 × 20	1 × 20	1 × 20	1 × 20	1 × 20	1 × 25	1 × 25
Hip hike	1 × 15	1 × 15	1 × 20	1 × 20	1 × 20	1 × 20	1 × 25	1 × 25
Hip hike (single leg)	1 × 15	1 × 15	1 × 15	1 × 20	1 × 20	1 × 20	1 × 20	1 × 20
V-up	1 × 15	1 × 15	1 × 15	2 × 15	2 × 20	2 × 20	2 × 20	2 × 20
Pillars					4 × :30	4 × :40	4 × :50	4 × :60
Pillars with partner resistance					1 × :20	2 × :20	2 × :30	2 × :30

Table 9.2   Abdominal and Core Program B (Advanced)

Week	1	2	3	4	5	6	7	8
Medicine ball: twist pass	2 × 30 (3 kg)	2 × 30 (3 kg)	2 × 30 (4 kg)	2 × 30 (4 kg)	2 × 30 (4 kg)	2 × 30 (4 kg)	2 × 30 (5 kg)	2 × 30 (5 kg)
Medicine ball: overhead throw	2 × 15 (3 kg)	2 × 15 (3 kg)	2 × 15 (4 kg)	2 × 15 (4 kg)	2 × 20 (4 kg)	2 × 20 (4 kg)	2 × 20 (5 kg)	2 × 20 (5 kg)
Medicine ball: side toss[a]	2 × 15 (3 kg)	2 × 15 (3 kg)	2 × 15 (4 kg)	2 × 15 (4 kg)	2 × 20 (4 kg)	2 × 20 (4 kg)	2 × 20 (5 kg)	2 × 20 (5 kg)
Medicine ball: bounce pass[b]	2 × 15 (3 kg)	2 × 15 (3 kg)	2 × 15 (4 kg)	2 × 15 (4 kg)	2 × 20 (4 kg)	2 × 20 (4 kg)	2 × 20 (5 kg)	2 × 20 (5 kg)
Elbow bridge	2 × 20	2 × 20	2 × 20	2 × 20	2 × 20	2 × 20	2 × 20	2 × 20
Bridge push-up	2 × 20	2 × 20	2 × 20	2 × 20	2 × 20	2 × 20	2 × 20	2 × 20
Hyperextension	1 × 20	1 × 20	1 × 20	1 × 20	1 × 25	1 × 25	1 × 25	1 × 25
Hip hike	1 × 20	1 × 20	1 × 20	1 × 20	1 × 25	1 × 25	1 × 25	1 × 25
Leg curl	2 × 10	2 × 10	2 × 10	2 × 10	2 × 15	2 × 15	2 × 15	2 × 15
Pike	1 × 15	1 × 15	1 × 15	1 × 15	1 × 15	1 × 15	1 × 15	1 × 15

[a] Medicine ball: side toss involves throwing the medicine ball to the side to a partner.

[b] Medicine ball: bounce pass (swing side) means throwing the medicine ball from your swing side down to bounce before a partner catches it.

Table 9.3　Speed Agility Preseason 6-Week Program

Group	Exercise	Page #	Volume
Daily six	High-knee skip	164	2 × 20 yd
	Heel kick	164	2 × 20 yd
	Straight-leg toe touch	165	2 × 20 yd
	Fast-feet: sideways	163	2 × 20 yd
	Forward–backward leg swing	159	2 × 20 yd
	Fast feet: backpedal	163	2 × 20 yd
Optional	Power skip	111	2 × 20 yd
	Carioca (crossover)	165	2 × 20 yd
	Backward stride	162	2 × 20 yd
Fast-feet drills	Fast-feet: forward	162	2 × 10 yd
	Fast-feet: forward, backward, forward	163	2 × 20 yd
Transition drills	Stop-and-go drill	117	4 × 6 cones (5 to 15 yd apart)
	Cutting drill	118	4 × 6 cones (5 to 15 yd apart)
	I-drill	119	5 sets
	Shuttle drill	119	5 sets
Main set drills—agility	Star drill	120	5 sets
	Two-foot barrier strides	115	1 × 4 ft, 1 × 5 ft, 1 × 6 ft
	Barrier strides	112	1 × 4 ft, 1 × 5 ft, 1 × 6 ft
Main set drills—running	Bounding	113	2 × 6 bounds
	Weighted sled towing	114	4 to 6 × 30 yd
	Downhill running	116	6 to 8 × 20 to 30 yd
	Bungee sprints	115	4 to 6 × 30 yd
	Slide board sprints	116	4 to 5 × 30 sec

1 foot = 0.3048 meters; 1 yard = 0.9144 meters

Off-Season 12-Week Program

Exercise	Page #	Weeks 1-4			Weeks 5-8			Weeks 9-12		
		Day 1	Day 2	Day 3	Day 1	Day 2	Day 3	Day 1	Day 2	Day 3
General strength										
Back squat or leg press	65 or 69	2 × 12 2 × 10		2 × 12 2 × 10	2 × 10 2 × 8		2 × 10 2 × 8	2 × 8 2 × 6		2 × 8 2 × 6
Bench press (incline)	55	2 × 12 2 × 10		2 × 12 2 × 10	2 × 10 2 × 8		2 × 10 2 × 8	2 × 8 2 × 6		2 × 8 2 × 6
Forward box step-up	73	1 × 12 1 × 10		1 × 12 1 × 10	1 × 10 1 × 8		1 × 10 1 × 8	1 × 8 1 × 6		1 × 8 1 × 6
Side box step-up	74	1 × 12 1 × 10		1 × 12 1 × 10	1 × 10 1 × 8		1 × 10 1 × 8	1 × 8 1 × 6		1 × 8 1 × 6
Lat pull-down	56	2 × 12 2 × 10		2 × 12 2 × 10	2 × 10 2 × 8		2 × 10 2 × 8	2 × 8 2 × 6		2 × 8 2 × 6
Walking lunge	72	3 × 12		3 × 12	3 × 15		3 × 15	3 × 20		3 × 20
Romanian deadlift	67	3 × 10		3 × 10	3 × 10		3 × 10	3 × 8		3 × 8
Shoulder press	55	3 × 10		3 × 10	3 × 8		3 × 8	3 × 6		3 × 6
Glute–ham: straight leg	71	1 × 15		1 × 15	1 × 15		1 × 15	2 × 15		2 × 15
Glute–ham: bent knee	92	1 × 15		1 × 15	2 × 15		2 × 15	2 × 15		2 × 15
General abs	169	Prog A		Prog A	Prog A		Prog A	Prog A		Prog A
Power										
Hang clean	127		2 × 6 2 × 5			2 × 5 2 × 4			2 × 4 2 × 3	
Push press	130		2 × 6 2 × 5			2 × 5 2 × 4			2 × 4 2 × 3	
Front squat	66		2 × 8 2 × 6			2 × 8 2 × 6			2 × 6 2 × 5	
High pull	126		2 × 6 2 × 5			2 × 5 2 × 4			2 × 4 2 × 3	
Squat jump	139		3 × 10			3 × 10			3 × 10	
Advanced abs	169		Prog B			Prog B			Prog B	

Choose only two of the three leg exercises on day 1 and day 3 (for example, squat and walking lunge).

For advanced abs, B program, choose three medicine ball exercises and three physioball exercises.

BASKETBALL

Preseason 6-Week Program

Exercise	Page #	Weeks 1-2			Weeks 3-4			Weeks 5-6		
		Day 1	Day 2	Day 3	Day 1	Day 2	Day 3	Day 1	Day 2	Day 3
General strength										
Back squat or leg press	65 or 69		2 × 6 2 × 5			2 × 6 2 × 5			2 × 6 2 × 5	
Bench press (incline)	55		2 × 6 2 × 5			2 × 6 2 × 5			2 × 6 2 × 5	
Forward box step-up	73		1 × 6 1 × 5			1 × 6 1 × 5			1 × 6 1 × 5	
Side box step-up	74		1 × 6 1 × 5			1 × 6 1 × 5			1 × 6 1 × 5	
Lat pull-down	56		2 × 6 2 × 5			2 × 6 2 × 5			2 × 6 2 × 5	
Romanian deadlift	67		2 × 10			2 × 10			2 × 10	
Shoulder press	55		3 × 6			3 × 5			3 × 5	
Glute–ham: straight leg	71		1 × 15			1 × 15			1 × 15	
Glute–ham: bent knee	92		2 × 15			2 × 15			2 × 15	
General abs	169		Prog A			Prog A			Prog A	
Power										
Hang clean	127	3 × 5		3 × 5	3 × 5		3 × 5	3 × 5		3 × 5
Push press	130	3 × 5		3 × 5	3 × 5		3 × 5	3 × 5		3 × 5
Front squat	66	3 × 5		3 × 5	3 × 5		3 × 5	3 × 5		3 × 5
High pull	126	3 × 5		3 × 5	3 × 5		3 × 5	3 × 5		3 × 5
Medicine ball: overhead throw	95	2 × 15		2 × 15	2 × 15		2 × 15	2 × 15		2 × 15
Medicine ball: chest pass	93	2 × 15		2 × 15	2 × 15		2 × 15	2 × 15		2 × 15
Medicine ball: twist pass	95	2 × 15		2 × 15	2 × 15		2 × 15	2 × 15		2 × 15
Extended crunch with pass	104	2 × 15		2 × 15	2 × 15		2 × 15	2 × 15		2 × 15

In-Season Maintenance 16-Week Program

Exercise	Page #	Weeks 1-16		
		Day 1	Day 2	Day 3
General strength				
Walking lunge	72		2 × 10	
Bench press (incline)	55		2 × 10	
Forward box step-up	73		1 × 10	
Side box step-up	74		1 × 10	
Lat pull-down	56		2 × 10	
Romanian deadlift	67		2 × 10	
Dumbbell rotator cuff routine (5 lb)	44		5 × 15	
Glute–ham: straight leg	71		1 × 15	
Glute–ham: bent knee	92		1 × 15	
General abs	169		Prog A	
Power				
Hang clean	127	3 × 5		O
Push press	130	3 × 5		P
Front squat	66	2 × 10		T
High pull	126	3 × 5		I
Walking lunge	72	2 × 15		O
Medicine ball: overhead throw	95	2 × 15		N
Medicine ball: chest pass	93	2 × 15		A
Medicine ball: twist pass	94	2 × 15		L
Extended crunch with pass	104	2 × 15		

Off-Season 12-Week Program

Exercise	Page #	Weeks 1-4			Weeks 5-8			Weeks 9-12		
		Day 1	Day 2	Day 3	Day 1	Day 2	Day 3	Day 1	Day 2	Day 3
General strength										
Back squat or leg press	65 or 69	2 × 12 1 × 10		2 × 12 1 × 10	2 × 10 1 × 8		2 × 10 1 × 8	2 × 8 2 × 6		2 × 8 2 × 6
Bench press	55	2 × 12 1 × 10		2 × 12 1 × 10	2 × 10 1 × 8		2 × 10 1 × 8	2 × 8 2 × 6		2 × 8 2 × 6
Forward box step-up	73	2 × 10		2 × 10	2 × 10		2 × 10	1 × 8 1 × 6		1 × 8 1 × 6
Side box step-up	74	1 × 10		1 × 10	1 × 10		1 × 10	1 × 8 1 × 6		1 × 8 1 × 6
Lat pull-down	56	2 × 12 1 × 10		2 × 12 1 × 10	2 × 10 1 × 8		2 × 10 1 × 8	2 × 8 2 × 6		2 × 8 2 × 6
Walking lunge	72	3 × 12		3 × 10	3 × 15		3 × 15	3 × 20		3 × 20
Handstand push-up	56	3 × 10		3 × 10	3 × 10		3 × 10			
Romanian deadlift	67	3 × 10		3 × 10	3 × 10		3 × 10	3 × 8		3 × 8
Dumbbell rotator cuff routine (5 lb or 2 kg)	44	5 × 10		5 × 10	5 × 12		5 × 12	5 × 15		5 × 15
Glute–ham: straight leg	71	1 × 15		1 × 15	2 × 15		2 × 15	2 × 15		4 × 15
Glute–ham: bent knee	92	1 × 15		1 × 15	1 × 15		1 × 15	2 × 15		2 × 15
General abs	169	Prog A		Prog A	Prog A		Prog A	Prog A		Prog A
Power										
Hang clean	127		2 × 6 2 × 5			2 × 5 2 × 4			2 × 4 2 × 3	
Push press	130		2 × 6 2 × 5			2 × 5 2 × 4			2 × 4 2 × 3	
High pull	126		2 × 6 2 × 5			2 × 5 2 × 4			2 × 4 2 × 3	
Side lunge	75		2 × 10			2 × 15			2 × 15	
Power push-up	55		3 × 8			3 × 10			3 × 12	
Medicine ball: twist pass	94		2 × 15			2 × 15			2 × 15	
Extended crunch with pass	104		2 × 15			2 × 15			2 × 15	
Bridge push-up	97		3 × 10			3 × 10			3 × 10	
Pike	98		2 × 10			2 × 12			3 × 15	
V-up	87		3 × 10			3 × 10			3 × 10	

Choose two of the three leg exercises on day 1 and day 3 (for example, squat and walking lunge).

Preseason 6-Week Program

Exercise	Page #	Weeks 1-2			Weeks 3-4			Weeks 5-6		
		Day 1	Day 2	Day 3	Day 1	Day 2	Day 3	Day 1	Day 2	Day 3
General strength										
Back squat or leg press	65 or 69	3 × 8		3 × 8	3 × 8		3 × 6	2 × 8 2 × 6		2 × 8 2 × 6
Bench press	55	3 × 8		3 × 8	3 × 8		3 × 6	2 × 8 2 × 6		2 × 8 2 × 6
Forward box step-up	73	2 × 8		2 × 8	2 × 8		2 × 6	1 × 8 1 × 6		1 × 8 1 × 6
Side box step-up	74	1 × 8		1 × 8	1 × 8		1 × 6	1 × 8 1 × 6		1 × 8 1 × 6
Lat pull-down	56	3 × 8		3 × 8	3 × 8		3 × 6	2 × 8 2 × 6		2 × 8 2 × 6
Walking lunge	72	3 × 12		3 × 12	3 × 12		3 × 12	3 × 20		3 × 20
Handstand push-up	56	3 × 10		3 × 10	3 × 10		3 × 10	3 × 10		3 × 10
Romanian deadlift	67	3 × 8		3 × 8	3 × 8		3 × 8	3 × 8		3 × 8
Dumbbell rotator cuff routine (5 lb or 2 kg)	44	5 × 10		5 × 10	5 × 10		5 × 12	5 × 15		5 × 15
Glute–ham: straight leg	71	2 × 15		2 × 15	2 × 15		2 × 15	2 × 15		2 × 15
Glute–ham: bent knee	92	2 × 15		2 × 15	2 × 15		2 × 15	2 × 15		2 × 15
General abs	169	Prog A		Prog A	Prog A		Prog A	Prog A		Prog A
Power										
Hang clean	127		3 × 5			3 × 5			3 × 4	
Push press	130		3 × 5			3 × 5			3 × 4	
High pull	126		3 × 5			3 × 5			3 × 4	
Tuck jump	136		3 × 8			3 × 8			3 × 8	
Power push-up	56		3 × 8			3 × 8			3 × 8	
Medicine ball: side toss	169		2 × 15			2 × 15			2 × 15	
Medicine ball: twist pass	94		2 × 15			2 × 15			2 × 15	
Extended crunch with pass	104		2 × 15			2 × 15			2 × 15	
Bridge push-up	97		3 × 10			3 × 10			3 × 10	
Pike	98		2 × 10			2 × 10			2 × 10	
Hanging knee raise	89		2 × 10			2 × 10			2 × 10	

In-Season Maintenance 16-Week Program

Exercise	Page #	Day 1	Day 2	Day 3
General strength				
Bench press (dumbbells)	55		2 × 10	
Forward box step-up	73		1 × 10	
Side box step-up	74		1 × 10	
Lat pull-down	56		2 × 10	
Walking lunge	72		2 × 10	
Handstand push-up	55		2 × 10	
Romanian deadlift	67		2 × 10	
Dumbbell rotator cuff routine (5 lb or 2 kg)	44		5 exercises × 15 each	
Glute–ham: straight leg	71		1 × 15	
Glute–ham: bent knee	92		1 × 15	
General abs	169		Prog A	
Power				
Pull-up	33	3 × 8		O
Push press	130	2 × 6		P
High pull	126	2 × 6		T
Tuck jump	136	2 × 8		I
Power push-up	56	3 × 8		O
Medicine ball: side toss	169	3 × 5		N
Medicine ball: twist pass	94	3 × 5		A
Extended crunch with pass	104	2 × 15		L
Bridge push-up	97	2 × 15		
Pike	98	2 × 15		
Hanging knee raise	89	2 × 15		

Off-Season 12-Week Program

Exercise	Page #	Weeks 1-4			Weeks 5-8			Weeks 9-12		
		Day 1	Day 2	Day 3	Day 1	Day 2	Day 3	Day 1	Day 2	Day 3
General strength										
Back squat or leg press	65 or 69	2 × 12 2 × 10		2 × 12 2 × 10	2 × 10 2 × 8		2 × 10 2 × 8	2 × 8 2 × 6		2 × 8 2 × 6
Bench press	55	2 × 12 2 × 10		2 × 12 2 × 10	2 × 10 2 × 8		2 × 10 2 × 8	2 × 8 2 × 6		2 × 8 2 × 6
Forward box step-up	73	1 × 12 1 × 10		1 × 12 1 × 10	1 × 10 1 × 8		1 × 10 1 × 8	1 × 8 1 × 6		1 × 8 1 × 6
Side box step-up	74	1 × 12 1 × 10		1 × 12 1 × 10	1 × 10 1 × 8		1 × 10 1 × 8	1 × 8 1 × 6		1 × 8 1 × 6
Lat pull-down	56	2 × 12 2 × 10		2 × 12 2 × 10	2 × 10 2 × 8		2 × 10 2 × 8	2 × 8 2 × 6		2 × 8 2 × 6
Walking lunge	72	3 × 12		3 × 12	3 × 15		3 × 15	3 × 20		3 × 20
Romanian deadlift	67	3 × 10		3 × 10	3 × 10		3 × 10	3 × 8		3 × 8
Dumbbell rotator cuff routine (5 lb or 2 kg)	44	5 × 10		5 × 10	5 × 12		5 × 12	5 × 15		5 × 15
Glute–ham: straight leg	71	1 × 15		1 × 15	2 × 15		2 × 15	2 × 15		2 × 15
Glute–ham: bent knee	92	1 × 15		1 × 15	1 × 15		1 × 15	2 × 15		2 × 15
General abs	169	Prog A		Prog A	Prog A		Prog A	Prog A		Prog A
Rice: three way	58	2 × 25		2 × 25	2 × 25		2 × 25	2 × 25		2 × 25
Power										
Hang clean	127		2 × 6 2 × 5			2 × 5 2 × 4			2 × 4 2 × 3	
Push press	130		2 × 6 2 × 5			2 × 5 2 × 4			2 × 4 2 × 3	
Squat jump	139		3 × 10			3 × 10			3 × 10	
High pull	126		2 × 6 2 × 5			2 × 5 2 × 4			2 × 4 2 × 3	
Side lunge	75		2 × 10			2 × 15			2 × 15	
Medicine ball: overhead throw	95		2 × 15			2 × 15			2 × 15	
Medicine ball: chest pass	93		2 × 15			2 × 15			2 × 15	
Medicine ball: twist pass	94		2 × 15			2 × 15			2 × 15	
Extended crunch with pass	104		2 × 15			2 × 15			2 × 15	
Rice: three way	58		3 × 25			3 × 35			3 × 45	

Choose two of the three leg exercises on day 1 and day 3 (for example, squat and walking lunge).

FIELD HOCKEY

Preseason 6-Week Program

Exercise	Page #	Weeks 1-2			Weeks 3-4			Weeks 5-6		
		Day 1	Day 2	Day 3	Day 1	Day 2	Day 3	Day 1	Day 2	Day 3
General strength										
Back squat or leg press	65 or 69		2 × 6 2 × 5			2 × 6 2 × 5			2 × 6 2 × 5	
Bench press	55		2 × 6 2 × 5			2 × 6 2 × 5			2 × 6 2 × 5	
Forward box step-up	73		1 × 6 1 × 5			1 × 6 1 × 5			1 × 6 1 × 5	
Side box step-up	74		1 × 6 1 × 5			1 × 6 1 × 5			1 × 6 1 × 5	
Lat pull-down	56		2 × 6 2 × 5			2 × 6 2 × 5			2 × 6 2 × 5	
Romanian deadlift	67		2 × 20			2 × 20			2 × 20	
Dumbbell rotator cuff routine (5 lb or 2 kg)	44		5 × 15			5 × 15			5 × 15	
Glute–ham: straight-leg	71		2 × 15			2 × 15			3 × 15	
Glute–ham: bent knee	92		1 × 15			1 × 15			1 × 15	
General abs	169		Prog A			Prog A			Prog A	
Rice: three way	58		3 × 25			3 × 25			3 × 25	
Power										
Hang clean	127	3 × 5		3 × 5	3 × 5		3 × 5	3 × 5		3 × 5
Push press	130	3 × 5		3 × 5	3 × 5		3 × 5	3 × 5		3 × 5
Squat jump	139	3 × 10		3 × 10	3 × 10		3 × 10	3 × 10		3 × 10
High pull	126	3 × 5		3 × 5	3 × 5		3 × 5	3 × 5		3 × 5
Advanced abs	169	Prog B		Prog B	Prog B		Prog B	Prog B		Prog B
Rice: three way	58	3 × 25		3 × 25	3 × 35		3 × 35	3 × 45		3 × 45

In-Season Maintenance 16-Week Program

Exercise	Page #	Weeks 1-16		
		Day 1	Day 2	Day 3
General strength				
Walking lunge	72		2 × 10	
Bench press	55		2 × 10	
Forward box step-up	73		1 × 10	
Side box step-up	74		1 × 10	
Lat pull-down	56		2 × 10	
Romanian deadlift	67		2 × 10	
Dumbbell rotator cuff routine (5 lb or 2 kg)	44		5 × 15	
Glute–ham: straight leg	71		1 × 15	
Glute–ham: bent knee	92		1 × 15	
General abs	169		Prog A	
Rice: three way	58		2 × 25	
Power				
Hang clean	127	3 × 5		O
Push press	130	3 × 5		P
High pull	126	3 × 5		T
Squat jump	139	3 × 10		I
Medicine ball: overhead throw	95	2 × 15		O
Medicine ball: chest pass	93	2 × 15		N
Medicine ball: twist pass	94	2 × 15		A
Extended crunch with pass	104	2 × 15		L

GOLF

Off-Season and Preseason 12-Week Program

Exercise	Page #	Weeks 1-4			Weeks 5-8			Weeks 9-12		
		Day 1	Day 2	Day 3	Day 1	Day 2	Day 3	Day 1	Day 2	Day 3
General strength										
Bench press	55	2 × 15	2 × 15	2 × 15	2 × 12	2 × 12	2 × 12	2 × 10	2 × 10	2 × 10
Leg press	69	2 × 15	2 × 15	2 × 15	2 × 12	2 × 12	2 × 12	2 × 10	2 × 10	2 × 10
Lat pull-down	56	2 × 15	2 × 15	2 × 15	2 × 12	2 × 12	2 × 12	2 × 10	2 × 10	2 × 10
Walking lunge	72	2 × 15	2 × 15	2 × 15	2 × 12	2 × 12	2 × 12	2 × 10	2 × 10	2 × 10
Seated row	57	2 × 15	2 × 15	2 × 15	2 × 12	2 × 12	2 × 12	2 × 10	2 × 10	2 × 10
Bungee swing	57	2 × 15	2 × 15	2 × 15	2 × 20	2 × 20	2 × 20	2 × 20	2 × 20	2 × 20
Dumbbell rotator cuff routine (3-5 lb or 1.5-2 kg)	44	5 × 10	5 × 10	5 × 10	5 × 12	5 × 12	5 × 12	2 × 12	2 × 12	2 × 12
Glute–ham: straight leg	71	2 × 15	2 × 15	2 × 15	2 × 15	2 × 15	2 × 15	2 × 15	2 × 15	2 × 15
Dumbbell take-away part of swing[a]	—	2 × 15	2 × 15	2 × 15	2 × 15	2 × 15	2 × 15	2 × 15	2 × 15	2 × 15
Dumbbell follow-through part of swing[b]	—	2 × 15	2 × 15	2 × 15	2 × 15	2 × 15	2 × 15	2 × 15	2 × 15	2 × 15
Core power										
Medicine ball: side toss (each side)	169	1 × 10	1 × 10	1 × 10	1 × 15	1 × 15	1 × 15	1 × 20	1 × 20	1 × 20
Medicine ball: bounce pass (swing side)	169	2 × 10	2 × 10	2 × 10	2 × 15	2 × 15	2 × 15	2 × 20	2 × 20	2 × 20
Medicine ball: twist (each side)	94	2 × 20	2 × 20	2 × 20	2 × 20	2 × 20	2 × 20	2 × 20	2 × 20	2 × 20
Medicine ball: chest pass	93	2 × 10	2 × 10	2 × 10	2 × 15	2 × 15	2 × 15	2 × 20	2 × 20	2 × 20
General abs and low back										
Bridge push-up	97	2 × 30	2 × 30	2 × 30	2 × 15	2 × 15	2 × 15	2 × 20	2 × 20	2 × 20
Hip hike	99	2 × 10	2 × 10	2 × 10	2 × 15	2 × 15	2 × 15	2 × 20	2 × 20	2 × 20
Hanging knee raise	89	2 × 10	2 × 10	2 × 10	2 × 15	2 × 15	2 × 15	2 × 20	2 × 20	2 × 20

Start each workout with the general abs routine (see pages 169). Take only 20 to 30 seconds between exercises. Complete a full circuit before repeating for the second set. For example, 2 × 12 means you should complete one set of 12 reps on your first circuit and complete your second set on the second circuit. Take two minutes of rest between circuits.

[a] Dumbbell take-away part of swing is performing the first part of swing using a dumbbell for resistance.

[b] Dumbbell follow-through part of swing is performing the second half of the swing using a dumbbell for resistance.

In-Season Maintenance Program

Exercise	Page #	Weeks 1 to 16		
		Day 1	Day 2	Day 3
General strength				
Bench press	55	2 × 8	2 × 8	O
Leg press	69	2 × 8	2 × 8	P
Lat pull-down	56	2 × 8	2 × 8	T
Walking lunge	72	2 × 8	2 × 8	I
Seated row	57	2 × 8	2 × 8	O
Bungee swing	57	2 × 15	2 × 15	N
Dumbbell rotator cuff routine (3-5 lb or 1.5-2 kg)	44	5 × 15	5 × 15	A
Glute–ham: straight leg	71	5 × 15	5 × 15	L
Dumbbell take-away part of swing[a]	—	5 × 15	5 × 15	
Dumbbell follow-through part of swing[b]	—	5 × 15	5 × 15	
Core power				
Medicine ball: side toss (each side)	169	2 × 15	2 × 15	O
Medicine ball: bounce pass (swing side)	169	2 × 15	2 × 15	P
Medicine ball: twist pass (each side)	94	2 × 15	2 × 15	T
Medicine ball: chest pass	93	2 × 15	2 × 15	O
General abs and low back				
Physioball swimmer	58	2 × 10	2 × 10	N
Hip hike	99	2 × 10	2 × 10	A
Hanging knee raise	89	2 × 10	2 × 10	L

[a] Dumbbell take-away part of swing is performing the first part of swing using a dumbbell for resistance.

[b] Dumbbell follow-through part of swing is performing the second half of the swing using a dumbbell for resistance.

GYMNASTICS

Off-Season 12-Week Program

Exercise	Page #	Weeks 1-4			Weeks 5-8			Weeks 9-12		
		Day 1	Day 2	Day 3	Day 1	Day 2	Day 3	Day 1	Day 2	Day 3
General strength										
Back squat or leg press	65 or 69	2 × 12 1 × 10		2 × 12 1 × 10	2 × 10 1 × 8		2 × 10 1 × 8	2 × 8 2 × 6		2 × 8 2 × 6
Bench press	55	2 × 12 1 × 10		2 × 12 1 × 10	2 × 10 1 × 8		2 × 10 1 × 8	2 × 8 2 × 6		2 × 8 2 × 6
Forward box step-up	73	2 × 10		2 × 10	2 × 10		2 × 10	1 × 8 1 × 6		1 × 8 1 × 6
Side box step-up	74	1 × 10		1 × 10	1 × 10		1 × 10	1 × 8 1 × 6		1 × 8 1 × 6
Lat pull-down	56	2 × 12 1 × 10		2 × 12 1 × 10	2 × 10 1 × 8		2 × 10 1 × 8	2 × 8 2 × 6		2 × 8 2 × 6
Walking lunge	72	3 × 12		3 × 10	3 × 15		3 × 15	3 × 20		3 × 20
Handstand push-up	56	3 × 10		3 × 10	3 × 10		3 × 10			
Romanian deadlift	67	3 × 10		3 × 10	3 × 10		3 × 10	3 × 8		3 × 8
Dumbbell rotator cuff routine (5 lb or 2 kg)	44	5 × 10		5 × 10	5 × 12		5 × 12	5 × 15		5 × 15
Glute–ham: straight leg	71	1 × 15		1 × 15	2 × 15		2 × 15	2 × 15		2 × 15
Glute–ham: bent knee	92	1 × 15		1 × 15	1 × 15		1 × 15	2 × 15		2 × 15
General abs	169	Prog A		Prog A	Prog A		Prog A	Prog A		Prog A
Power										
Squat jump	139		3 × 8			3 × 8			3 × 8	
Hang clean	127		2 × 6 2 × 5			2 × 5 2 × 4			2 × 4 2 × 3	
Side lunge	75		3 × 8			3 × 10			3 × 12	
Push press	130		2 × 6 2 × 5			2 × 5 2 × 4			2 × 4 2 × 3	
Diagonal skating	117		2 × 10			2 × 10			2 × 12	
Medicine ball: side toss	169		2 × 15			2 × 15			2 × 15	
Medicine ball: twist pass	94		2 × 15			2 × 15			2 × 15	
Extended crunch with pass	104		2 × 15			2 × 15			2 × 15	
Bridge push-up	97		3 × 10			3 × 10			3 × 10	
Pike	98		2 × 10			2 × 12			3 × 15	
V-up	87		3 × 10			3 × 10			3 × 10	

Choose two of the three leg exercises on day 1 and day 3 (for example, squat and walking lunge).

Preseason 6-Week Program

Exercise	Page #	Weeks 1-2			Weeks 3-4			Weeks 5-6		
		Day 1	Day 2	Day 3	Day 1	Day 2	Day 3	Day 1	Day 2	Day 3
Back squat or leg press	65 or 69	3 × 8		3 × 8	3 × 8		3 × 6	2 × 8 2 × 6		2 × 8 2 × 6
Bench press	55	3 × 8		3 × 8	3 × 8		3 × 6	2 × 8 2 × 6		2 × 8 2 × 6
Forward box step-up	73	3 × 8		3 × 8	3 × 8		3 × 6	1 × 8 1 × 6		1 × 8 1 × 6
Side box step-up	74	1 × 8		1 × 8	1 × 8		1 × 6	1 × 8 1 × 6		1 × 8 1 × 6
Pull-up	33	3 × 8		3 × 8	3 × 8		3 × 6	2 × 8 2 × 6		2 × 8 2 × 6
Walking lunge	72	3 × 12		3 × 12	3 × 12		3 × 12	3 × 20		3 × 20
Handstand push-up	56	3 × 10		3 × 10	3 × 10		3 × 10	3 × 10		3 × 10
Romanian deadlift	67	3 × 8		3 × 8	3 × 8		3 × 8	3 × 8		3 × 8
Dumbbell rotator cuff routine (5 lb or 2 kg)	44	5 × 10		5 × 10	5 × 10		5 × 12	5 × 15		5 × 15
Glute–ham: straight leg	71	4 × 15		4 × 15	4 × 15		4 × 15	4 × 15		4 × 15
Glute–ham: bent knee	92	2 × 15		2 × 15	2 × 15		2 × 15	2 × 15		2 × 15
General abs	169	Prog A		Prog A	Prog A		Prog A	Prog A		Prog A
Power										
Hang clean	127		3 × 5			3 × 5			3 × 4	
Push press	130		3 × 5			3 × 5			3 × 4	
Squat jump	139		3 × 8			3 × 8			3 × 8	
High pull	126		3 × 5			3 × 5			3 × 4	
Tuck jump	136		3 × 8			3 × 8			3 × 8	
Medicine ball: side toss	169		2 × 15			2 × 15			2 × 15	
Medicine ball: twist pass	94		2 × 15			2 × 15			2 × 15	
Extended crunch with pass	104		2 × 15			2 × 15			2 × 15	
Bridge push-up	97		3 × 10			3 × 10			3 × 10	
Hip hike	99		2 × 10			2 × 12			3 × 15	
Hanging knee raise	89		2 × 10			2 × 10			2 × 10	
V-up	87		3 × 10			3 × 10			3 × 10	

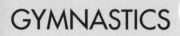
In-Season Maintenance 16-Week Program

Exercise	Page #	Weeks 1-16		
		Day 1	Day 2	Day 3
General strength				
Bench press (dumbbell)	55		2 × 10	
Forward box step-up	73		1 × 10	
Side box step-up	74		1 × 10	
Pull-up	33		2 ×10	
Walking lunge	72		2 × 10	
Handstand push-up	56		2 × 10	
Romanian deadlift	67		2 × 10	
Dumbbell rotator cuff routine (5 lb or 2 kg)	44		5 × 15	
Glute–ham: straight leg	71		1 × 15	
Glute–ham: bent knee	92		1 × 15	
General abs	169		Prog A	
Power				
Push press	130	2 × 6		O
High pull	126	2 × 6		P
Power push-up	56	3 × 8		T
Tuck jump	136	2 × 8		I
Medicine ball: chest pass	93	3 × 5		O
Medicine ball: twist pass	94	3 × 5		N
Extended crunch with pass	104	2 × 15		A
Bridge push-up	97	2 × 15		L
Hip hike	99	2 × 15		
Hanging knee raise	89	2 × 15		
V-up	87	2 × 15		

Off-Season 12-Week Program

Exercise	Page #	Weeks 1-4			Weeks 5-8			Weeks 9-12		
		Day 1	Day 2	Day 3	Day 1	Day 2	Day 3	Day 1	Day 2	Day 3
General strength										
Back squat or leg press	65 or 69	2 × 12 2 × 10		2 × 12 2 × 10	2 × 10 2 × 8		2 × 10 2 × 8	2 × 8 2 × 6		2 × 8 2 × 6
Bench press	55	2 × 12 2 × 10		2 × 12 2 × 10	2 × 10 2 × 8		2 × 10 2 × 8	2 × 8 2 × 6		2 × 8 2 × 6
Forward box step-up	73	1 × 12 1 × 10		1 × 12 1 × 10	1 × 10 1 × 8		1 × 10 1 × 8	1 × 8 1 × 6		1 × 8 1 × 6
Side box step-up	74	1 × 12 1 × 10		1 × 12 1 × 10	1 × 10 1 × 8		1 × 10 1 × 8	1 × 8 1 × 6		1 × 8 1 × 6
Lat pull-down	56	2 × 12 2 × 10		2 × 12 2 × 10	2 × 10 2 × 8		2 × 10 2 × 8	2 × 8 2 × 6		2 × 8 2 × 6
Walking lunge	72	3 × 12		3 × 12	3 × 15		3 × 15	3 × 20		3 × 20
Romanian deadlift	67	3 × 10		3 × 10	3 × 10		3 × 10	3 × 8		3 × 8
Dumbbell rotator cuff routine (5 lb or 2 kg)	44	5 × 10		5 × 10	5 × 12		5 × 12	5 × 15		5 × 15
Glute–ham: straight leg	71	1 × 15		1 × 15	2 × 15		2 × 15	2 × 15		2 × 15
Glute–ham: bent knee	92	1 × 15		1 × 15	1 × 15		1 × 15	2 × 15		2 × 15
General abs	169	Prog A		Prog A	Prog A		Prog A	Prog A		Prog A
Rice: three way	58	2 × 25		2 × 25	2 × 25		2 × 25	2 × 25		2 × 25
Power										
Hang clean	127		2 × 6 2 × 5			2 × 5 2 × 4			2 × 4 2 × 3	
Push press	130		2 × 6 2 × 5			2 × 5 2 × 4			2 × 4 2 × 3	
Side lunge	75		2 × 10			2 × 15			2 × 15	
High pull	126		2 × 6 2 × 5			2 × 5 2 × 4			2 × 4 2 × 3	
Medicine ball: overhead throw	95		2 × 15			2 × 15			2 × 15	
Medicine ball: chest pass	93		2 × 15			2 × 15			2 × 15	
Medicine ball: twist pass	94		2 × 15			2 × 15			2 × 15	
Extended crunch with pass	104		2 × 15			2 × 15			2 × 15	

Choose two of the three leg exercises on day 1 and day 3 (for example, squat and walking lunge).

LACROSSE

Preseason 6-Week Program

Exercise	Page #	Weeks 1-2			Weeks 3-4			Weeks 5-6		
		Day 1	Day 2	Day 3	Day 1	Day 2	Day 3	Day 1	Day 2	Day 3
General strength										
Back squat or leg press	65 or 69		2 × 6 2 × 5			2 × 6 2 × 5			2 × 6 2 × 5	
Bench press	55		2 × 6 2 × 5			2 × 6 2 × 5			2 × 6 2 × 5	
Forward box step-up	73		1 × 6 1 × 5			1 × 6 1 × 5			1 × 6 1 × 5	
Side box step-up	74		1 × 6 1 × 5			1 × 6 1 × 5			1 × 6 1 × 5	
Lat pull-down	56		2 × 6 2 × 5			2 × 6 2 × 5			2 × 6 2 × 5	
Romanian deadlift	67		2 × 20			2 × 20			2 × 20	
Rotator cuff routine (5 lb or 2 kg)	44		5 × 15			5 × 15			5 × 15	
Glute–ham: straight leg	71		2 × 15			2 × 15			2 × 15	
Glute–ham: bent knee	92		1 × 15			1 × 15			1 × 15	
General abs	169		Prog A			Prog A			Prog A	
Rice: three way	58		2 × 25			2 × 25			2 × 25	
Power										
Hang clean	127	3 × 5		3 × 5	3 × 5		3 × 5	3 × 5		3 × 5
Push press	130	3 × 5		3 × 5	3 × 5		3 × 5	3 × 5		3 × 5
High pull	126	3 × 5		3 × 5	3 × 5		3 × 5	3 × 5		3 × 5
Advanced abs	169	Prog B		Prog B	Prog B		Prog B	Prog B		Prog B

In-Season Maintenance 16-Week Program

Exercise	Page #	Weeks 1-16		
		Day 1	Day 2	Day 3
General strength				
Walking lunge	72		2 × 10	
Bench press	55		2 × 10	
Forward box step-up	73		1 × 10	
Side box step-up	74		1 × 10	
Lat pull-down	56		2 × 10	
Romanian deadlift	67		2 × 10	
Dumbbell rotator cuff routine (5 lb or 2 kg)	44		5 × 15	
Glute–ham: straight leg	71		1 × 15	
Glute–ham: bent knee	92		1 × 15	
General abs	169		Prog A	
Rice: three way	58		2 × 25	
Power				O
Hang clean	127	3 × 5		P
Push press	130	3 × 5		T
High pull	126	3 × 5		I
Medicine ball: overhead throw	95	2 × 15		O
Medicine ball: chest pass	93	2 × 15		N
Medicine ball: twist pass	94	2 × 15		A
Extended crunch with pass	104	2 × 15		L

Off-Season 12-Week Program

Exercise	Page #	Weeks 1-4			Weeks 5-8			Weeks 9-12		
		Day 1	Day 2	Day 3	Day 1	Day 2	Day 3	Day 1	Day 2	Day 3
General strength										
Back squat	65	2 × 12 2 × 10		2 × 12 2 × 10	2 × 10 2 × 8		2 × 10 2 × 8	2 × 8 2 × 6		2 × 8 2 × 6
Bench press	52	2 × 12 2 × 10		2 × 12 2 × 10	2 × 10 2 × 8		2 × 10 2 × 8	2 × 8 2 × 6		2 × 8 2 × 6
Forward box step-up	73	1 × 12 1 × 10		1 × 12 1 × 10	1 × 10 1 × 8		1 × 10 1 × 8	1 × 8 1 × 6		1 × 8 1 × 6
Side box step-up	74	1 × 12 1 × 10		1 × 12 1 × 10	1 × 10 1 × 8		1 × 10 1 × 8	1 × 8 1 × 6		1 × 8 1 × 6
Lat pull-down	56	2 × 12 2 × 10		2 × 12 2 × 10	2 × 10 2 × 8		2 × 10 2 × 8	2 × 8 2 × 6		2 × 8 2 × 6
Walking lunge	72	3 × 12		3 × 12	3 × 15		3 × 15	3 × 20		3 × 20
Romanian deadlift	67	3 × 10		3 × 10	3 × 10		3 × 10	3 × 8		3 × 8
Dumbbell rotator cuff routine (5 lb or 2 kg)	44	5 × 10		5 × 10	5 × 12		5 × 12	5 × 15		5 × 15
Glute–ham: straight leg	71	1 × 15		1 × 15	2 × 15		2 × 15	2 × 15		2 × 15
Glute–ham: bent knee	92	1 × 15		1 × 15	1 × 15		1 × 15	2 × 15		2 × 15
General abs	169	Prog A		Prog A	Prog A		Prog A	Prog A		Prog A
Power										
Hang clean	127		2 × 6 2 × 5			2 × 5 2 × 4			2 × 4 2 × 3	
Push press	130		2 × 6 2 × 5			2 × 5 2 × 4			2 × 4 2 × 3	
High pull	126		2 × 6 2 × 5			2 × 5 2 × 4			2 × 4 2 × 3	
Three-way weight transfer	76		1 × 10 each			1 × 15 each			1 × 15 each	
Side lunge	75		2 × 10			2 × 15			2 × 15	
Medicine ball: overhead throw	95		2 × 15			2 × 15			2 × 15	
Medicine ball: chest pass	93		2 × 15			2 × 15			2 × 15	
Medicine ball: twist pass	94		2 × 15			2 × 15			2 × 15	
Extended crunch with pass	104		2 × 15			2 × 15			2 × 15	

Choose two of the three leg exercises on day 1 and day 3 (for example, squat and walking lunge).

Preseason 6-Week Program

Exercise	Page #	Weeks 1-2			Weeks 3-4			Weeks 5-6		
		Day 1	Day 2	Day 3	Day 1	Day 2	Day 3	Day 1	Day 2	Day 3
General strength										
Back squat	65		2 × 6 2 × 5			2 × 6 2 × 5			2 × 6 2 × 5	
Bench press	55		2 × 6 2 × 5			2 × 6 2 × 5			2 × 6 2 × 5	
Forward box step-up	73		1 × 6 1 × 5			1 × 6 1 × 5			1 × 6 1 × 5	
Side box step-up	74		1 × 6 1 × 5			1 × 6 1 × 5			1 × 6 1 × 5	
Lat pull-down	56		2 × 6 2 × 5			2 × 6 2 × 5			2 × 6 2 × 5	
Romanian deadlift	67		2 × 10			2 × 10			2 × 10	
Dumbbell rotator cuff routine (5 lb or 2 kg)	44		5 × 15			5 × 15			5 × 15	
Glute–ham: straight leg	71		2 × 15			2 × 15			2 × 15	
Glute–ham: bent knee	92		1 × 15			1 × 15			1 × 15	
General abs	169		Prog A			Prog A			Prog A	
Power										
Hang clean	127	3 × 5		3 × 5	3 × 5		3 × 5	3 × 5		3 × 5
Push press	130	3 × 5		3 × 5	3 × 5		3 × 5	3 × 5		3 × 5
Side lunge	75	2 × 10		2 × 10	2 × 10		2 × 10	2 × 10		2 × 10
High pull	126	3 × 5		3 × 5	3 × 5		3 × 5	3 × 5		3 × 5
Medicine ball: overhead throw	95	2 × 15		2 × 15	2 × 15		2 × 15	2 × 15		2 × 15
Medicine ball: chest pass	93	2 × 15		2 × 15	2 × 15		2 × 15	2 × 15		2 × 15
Medicine ball: twist pass	94	2 × 15		2 × 15	2 × 15		2 × 15	2 × 15		2 × 15
Extended crunch with pass	104	2 × 15		2 × 15	2 × 15		2 × 15	2 × 15		2 × 15

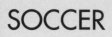

SOCCER

In-Season Maintenance 16-Week Program

Exercise	Page #	Weeks 1-16 Day 1	Weeks 1-16 Day 2	Weeks 1-16 Day 3
General strength				
Back squat	65		2 × 10	
Bench press	55		2 × 10	
Forward box step-up	73		1 × 10	
Side box step-up	74		1 × 10	
Lat pull-down	56		2 × 10	
Romanian deadlift	67		2 × 10	
Dumbbell rotator cuff routine (5 lb or 2 kg)	44		5 × 15	
Glute–ham: straight leg	71		1 × 15	
Glute–ham: bent knee	92		1 × 15	
General abs	169		Prog A	
Power				
Hang clean	127	3 × 5		O
Push press	130	3 × 5		P
High pull	126	3 × 5		T
Walking lunge	72	2 × 15		I
Medicine ball: overhead throw	95	2 × 15		O
Medicine ball: chest pass	93	2 × 15		N
Medicine ball: twist pass	94	2 × 15		A
Extended crunch with pass	104	2 × 15		L

Off-Season 12-Week Program—Weeks 1 Through 4

Exercise	Page #	Monday 1	Monday 2	Monday 3	Monday 4	Wednesday 1	Wednesday 2	Wednesday 3	Wednesday 4	Friday 1	Friday 2	Friday 3	Friday 4
Back squat	65	3 × 8	3 × 10	4 × 10	3 × 8								
Walking lunge	72	3 × 12	3 × 12	3 × 12	2 × 12								
Forward box step-up	73	3 × 12	4 × 12	4 × 12	2 × 12								
Lat pull-down	56	3 × 12	3 × 10	3 × 10	2 × 10								
Dumbbell rotator cuff routine	44	1 × 10	1 × 10	1 × 10	1 × 10					1 × 10	1 × 10	1 × 10	1 × 10
Body-weight shoulder stabilization routine	49	2 × 10	2 × 10	2 × 10	2 × 10	2 × 10	2 × 10	2 × 10	1 × 10				
Reverse hyper-extension	101					3 × 8	3 × 10	3 × 12	2 × 12				
Traditional deadlift	68					3 × 8	3 × 8	3 × 10	2 × 10				
Bench press (dumbbell)	55					3 × 10	3 × 12	3 × 12	2 × 10				
Seated row	57					3 × 12	3 × 12	3 × 12	3 × 8				
Front squat	66									3 × 10	4 × 10	4 × 10	2 × 10
Romanian deadlift	67									3 × 10	3 × 10	4 × 10	2 × 10
Side lunge	75									3 × 12	4 × 12	4 × 12	2 × 12
Bench press (incline)	55									3 × 10	3 × 12	3 × 12	2 × 10
General abs	169	Prog A	Prog A	Prog A	Prog A					Prog A	Prog A	Prog A	Prog A
Advanced abs	169	Prog B	Prog B	Prog B	Prog B					Prog B	Prog B	Prog B	Prog B
Jump rope drills	124					1 set	1-2 sets	2 sets	2 sets				

Off-Season 12-Week Program—Weeks 5 Through 8

Exercise	Page #	Monday 1	Monday 2	Monday 3	Monday 4	Wednesday 1	Wednesday 2	Wednesday 3	Wednesday 4	Friday 1	Friday 2	Friday 3	Friday 4
Power shrug	125	3 × 4	3 × 4	3 × 3	3 × 3								
High pull	126	3 × 3	3 × 3	3 × 3									
Hang clean	127	3 × 6	4 × 6	4 × 5	5RM	4 × 4	4 × 4	4 × 3	3RM				
Back squat	65	4 × 8	4 × 6	4 × 5	5RM								
Shoulder press (standing)	55	4 × 8	4 × 6	4 × 5	5RM								
Dumbbell rotator cuff routine	44	1 × 10	1 × 10	1 × 10	1 × 10								
Body-weight shoulder stabilization routine	49					2 × 10	2 × 10	2 × 10	2 × 10				
Front squat	66					4 × 8	4 × 6	4 × 5	5RM				
Romanian deadlift	67					4 × 8	4 × 8	4 × 8	2 × 8				
Seated row	57					3 × 10	3 × 10	3 × 10	2 × 10				
Glute–ham: straight leg	71					3 × 12	3 × 12	3 × 15	2 × 12				
Power clean	129									3 × 6	4 × 5	4 × 5	5RM
High pull	126									3 × 3	3 × 3	3 × 3	3 × 3
Bench press (incline)	55									3 × 8	4 × 8	4 × 8	6RM
Lat pull-down	56									3 × 10	3 × 10	3 × 10	2 × 10
Glute–ham: bent knee	92									3 × 10	3 × 10	3 × 10	2 × 10
Side box step-up	74									3 × 12	3 × 12	3 × 12	2 × 12
General abs	169	Prog A	Prog A	Prog A	Prog A					Prog A	Prog A	Prog A	Prog A
Advanced abs	169					Prog B	Prog B	Prog B	Prog B				
Low-intensity plyometrics	133	1-2 sets	2 sets	2 sets	1 set					1-2 sets	2 sets	2 sets	1 set

Off-Season 12-Week Program—Weeks 9 Through 12

Exercise	Page #	Monday 1	Monday 2	Monday 3	Monday 4	Wednesday 1	Wednesday 2	Wednesday 3	Wednesday 4	Friday 1	Friday 2	Friday 3	Friday 4
Power shrug	125	3 × 4	3 × 4	3 × 3	3 × 3								
Power clean	129	4 × 4	5 × 4	5 × 3	3RM					4 × 5	5 × 4	5 × 3	3 × 3
Back squat	65	4 × 6	5 × 5	4 × 4	3RM								
Shoulder press (standing)	55	4 × 6	4 × 5	4 × 4	3 × 4								
Lat pull-down	56	3 × 8	3 × 8	3 × 8	2 × 8								
Hang clean	127					4 × 4	4 × 3	4 × 3	3 × 3				
Traditional deadlift	68					4 × 6	4 × 6	4 × 6	2 × 6				
Bench press	55					4 × 5	4 × 4	4 × 3	3RM				
Seated row	57					4 × 8	4 × 8	4 × 8	2 × 8				
Glute–ham: straight leg	71					3 × 12	3 × 12	3 × 15	2 × 12				
Front squat	66									4 × 6	4 × 5	4 × 5	5RM
Side lunge	75									4 × 12	4 × 12	4 × 12	3 × 12
Bench press (incline)	55									4 × 8	4 × 6	4 × 5	2 × 5
Glute–ham: bent knee	92									3 × 10	3 × 10	3 × 10	2 × 10
General abs	169	Prog A	Prog A	Prog A	Prog A					Prog A	Prog A	Prog A	Prog A
Advanced abs	169					Prog B	Prog B	Prog B	Prog B				
Low-intensity plyometrics	133									1-2 sets	2 sets	2 sets	1 set
Moderate-intensity plyometrics	136	1-2 sets	2 sets	2 sets	1 set								

Preseason 12-Week Program—Weeks 1 Through 4

Exercise	Page #	Monday 1	Monday 2	Monday 3	Monday 4	Wednesday 1	Wednesday 2	Wednesday 3	Wednesday 4	Friday 1	Friday 2	Friday 3	Friday 4
Power shrug	125	3 × 4	3 × 4	3 × 4	2 × 3								
Hang clean	127	3 × 5	3 × 4	3 × 4	2 × 4					4 × 4	4 × 3	4 × 3	2 × 2
Front squat	66	3 × 6	4 × 6	4 × 5	2 × 5								
Side lunge	75	3 × 12	3 × 12	3 × 12	2 × 12								
Dumbbell rotator cuff routine	44	1 × 10	1 × 10	1 × 10	1 × 10					1 × 10	1 × 10	1 × 10	1 × 10
Body-weight shoulder stabilization routine	49					2 × 10	2 × 10	2 × 10	1 × 10				
High pull	126					3 × 4	3 × 4	3 × 4	2 × 3				
Power clean	129					3 × 4	3 × 4	3 × 3	2 × 3				
Bench press	55					3 × 6	3 × 6	3 × 6	2 × 6				
Lat pull-down	56					3 × 10	3 × 10	3 × 10	2 × 10				
Bench press (dumbbell, incline)	55					3 × 6	3 × 6	3 × 6	2 × 6				
Back squat	65									3 × 6	4 × 6	4 × 6	2 × 6
Forward box step-up	73									3 × 12	4 × 12	4 × 12	2 × 12
Glute–ham: bent knee	92									3 × 10	3 × 12	3 × 12	2 × 10
Side box step-up	74									3 × 12	4 × 12	4 × 12	2 × 12
General abs	169	Prog A	Prog A	Prog A	Prog A					Prog A	Prog A	Prog A	Prog A
Advanced abs	169	Prog B	Prog B	Prog B	Prog B					Prog B	Prog B	Prog B	Prog B
Jump rope drills	124					1 set	1-2 sets	2 sets	2 sets				

Preseason 12-Week Program—Weeks 5 Through 8

Exercise	Page #	Monday 1	2	3	4	Wednesday 1	2	3	4	Friday 1	2	3	4
Power shrug	125	3 × 4	3 × 4	3 × 4	2 × 3								
High pull	126	3 × 5	3 × 4	3 × 4	2 × 4					4 × 4	4 × 3	4 × 3	2 × 2
Power clean	129	4 × 3	5 × 3	5 × 3	2 × 3					4 × 3	5 × 2	5 × 2	2 × 2
Front squat	66	4 × 5	4 × 5	4 × 4	2 × 4								
Romanian deadlift	67	3 × 10	3 × 10	3 × 8	2 × 8								
Dumbbell rotator cuff routine	44	1 × 10	1 × 10	1 × 10	1 × 10					1 × 10	1 × 10	1 × 10	1 × 10
Body-weight shoulder stabilization routine	49					2 × 10	2 × 10	2 × 10	1 × 10				
Hang clean	127					4 × 3	5 × 2	5 × 2	3 × 3				
Bench press	55					3 × 6	3 × 5	3 × 5	5RM				
Shoulder press (seated)	55					3 × 10	3 × 8	3 × 8	2 × 8				
Lat pull-down	56					3 × 10	3 × 10	3 × 8	2 × 8				
Bench press (dumbbell, incline)	55					3 × 6	3 × 6	3 × 6	2 × 6				
Back squat	65									4 × 5	4 × 5	4 × 4	2 × 4
Forward box step-up	73									3 × 12	4 × 12	4 × 12	2 × 12
Glute–ham: bent knee	92									3 × 10	3 × 8	3 × 8	2 × 8
Side lunge	75									3 × 12	4 × 12	4 × 12	2 × 12
General abs	169	Prog A	Prog A	Prog A	Prog A					Prog A	Prog A	Prog A	Prog A
Advanced abs	169					Prog B	Prog B	Prog B	Prog B				
Low-intensity plyometrics	133	1-2 sets	2 sets	2 sets	1 set					1-2 sets	2 sets	2 sets	1 set

Preseason 12-Week Program—Weeks 9 Through 12

Exercise	Page #	Monday 1	Monday 2	Monday 3	Monday 4	Wednesday 1	Wednesday 2	Wednesday 3	Wednesday 4	Friday 1	Friday 2	Friday 3	Friday 4
Power shrug	125	3 × 4	3 × 4	3 × 4	2 × 3								
High pull	126	3 × 5	3 × 4	3 × 4	2 × 4					3 × 3	3 × 3	3 × 3	
Power clean	129	4 × 3	5 × 2	5 × 1	1RM					4 × 2	5 × 2	5 × 2	
Front squat	66	4 × 4	4 × 3	4 × 3	3RM								
Romanian deadlift	67	3 × 8	3 × 8	3 × 8									
Dumbbell rotator cuff routine	44	1 × 10	1 × 10	1 × 10	1 × 10					1 × 10	1 × 10	1 × 10	1 × 10
Body-weight shoulder stabilization routine	49					2 × 10	2 × 10	2 × 10	1 × 10				
Hang clean	127					4 × 2	5 × 2	5 × 1	1RM				
Bench press	55					3 × 4	3 × 3	3 × 3	3RM				
Shoulder press (seated)	55					3 × 8	3 × 8	3 × 8	2 × 10				
Lat pull-down	56					3 × 10	3 × 8	3 × 8	2 × 8				
Bench press (dumbbell, incline)	55					2 × 6	2 × 6	2 × 6					
Back squat	65									4 × 3	5 × 2	4 × 2	1RM
Forward box step-up	73									3 × 12	3 × 12	3 × 12	2 × 12
Glute–ham: bent knee	92									3 × 10	3 × 8	3 × 8	2 × 8
Side lunge	75									3 × 12	3 × 12	3 × 12	2 × 12
General abs	169	Prog A	Prog A	Prog A	Prog A					Prog A	Prog A	Prog A	Prog A
Low-intensity plyometrics	133									1-2 sets	2 sets	2 sets	1 set
Moderate-intensity plyometrics	136	1-2 sets	2 sets	2 sets	1 set								

In-Season Maintenance 12-Week Program—Weeks 1 Through 12

Exercise	Page #	Monday				Wednesday				Friday			
		1	2	3	4	1	2	3	4	1	2	3	4
Power shrug	125	2 × 4	2 × 4	2 × 4	2 × 3								
High pull	126	2 × 3	2 × 3	2 × 3	2 × 3					2 × 3	2 × 3	2 × 3	2 × 3
Power clean	129	3 × 3	4 × 2	3 × 3	2 × 2					3 × 3	4 × 2	3 × 3	2 × 2
Front squat	66	3 × 5	3 × 4	3 × 3	2 × 4								
Romanian deadlift	67	2 × 8	2 × 8	2 × 8									
Dumbbell rotator cuff routine	44	1 × 10	1 × 10	1 × 10	1 × 10					1 × 10	1 × 10	1 × 10	1 × 10
Body-weight shoulder stabilization routine	49					2 × 10	2 × 10	2 × 10	1 × 10				
Hang clean	127					3 × 3	4 × 2	3 × 3	2 × 2				
Bench press	55					2 × 6	2 × 5	2 × 6	2 × 5				
Lat pull-down	56					2 × 8	3 × 8	2 × 8	2 × 8				
Bench press (dumbbell, incline)	55					2 × 6	2 × 6	2 × 6					
Back squat	65									3 × 6	3 × 5	3 × 4	2 × 6
Forward box step-up	73									2 × 12	3 × 12	2 × 12	2 × 12
Glute–ham: bent knee	92									2 × 10	2 × 8	3 × 8	
Side lunge	75									2 × 12	3 × 12	2 × 12	2 × 12
General abs	169	Prog A	Prog A	Prog A	Prog A					Prog A	Prog A	Prog A	Prog A
Low-intensity plyometrics	133									1-2 sets	2 sets	2 sets	1 set
Moderate-intensity plyometrics	136	1-2 sets	2 sets	2 sets	1 set								

Off-Season 12-Week Program—Weeks 1 Through 4

Exercise	Page #	Monday 1	2	3	4	Wednesday 1	2	3	4	Friday 1	2	3	4
Back squat	65	4 × 12	4 × 10	4 × 8	3 × 8								
Shoulder press (standing)	55	4 × 12	4 × 10	4 × 10	2 × 10					4 × 12	4 × 10	4 × 8	3 × 8
Walking lunge	72	3 × 12	3 × 12	3 × 12	2 × 12								
Forward box step-up	73	4 × 12	4 × 12	4 × 12	2 × 12								
Lat pull-down	56	3 × 12	3 × 10	3 × 10	2 × 10								
Standing two-way calf raise	77	3 × 12	3 × 12	3 × 12	2 × 12								
Traditional deadlift	68					4 × 12	4 × 10	4 × 8	3 × 8				
Push press	130					4 × 10	4 × 8	4 × 6	3 × 6				
Single-leg knee extension	70					4 × 12	4 × 12	4 × 10	2 × 10				
Glute–ham: straight leg	71					3 × 10	3 × 12	3 × 15	2 × 15				
Dumbbell rotator cuff routine	44					5 × 10	5 × 10	3 × 12	3 × 12				
Seated row	57					3 × 12	3 × 12	3 × 10	3 × 8	4 × 12	4 × 10	4 × 8	3 × 8
Front squat	66									4 × 10	4 × 10	4 × 10	2 × 10
Romanian deadlift	67									3 × 10	3 × 10	4 × 10	2 × 10
Bench press	55									4 × 12	4 × 10	4 × 8	3 × 8
General abs	169	Prog A	Prog A	Prog A	Prog A					Prog A	Prog A	Prog A	Prog A
Advanced abs	169	Prog B	Prog B	Prog B	Prog B					Prog B	Prog B	Prog B	Prog B
Jump rope drills	124					1 set	1-2 sets	2 sets	2 sets				

198

Off-Season 12-Week Program—Weeks 5 Through 8

Exercise	Page #	Monday 1	Monday 2	Monday 3	Monday 4	Wednesday 1	Wednesday 2	Wednesday 3	Wednesday 4	Friday 1	Friday 2	Friday 3	Friday 4
Power shrug	125	3 × 4	3 × 4	3 × 3	3 × 3					3 × 3	3 × 3	3 × 3	3 × 3
Hang clean	127	4 × 6	4 × 6	4 × 5	5RM	4 × 4	4 × 4	4 × 3	3 × 3				
High pull	126	3 × 3	3 × 3	3 × 3									
Back squat	65	4 × 8	4 × 6	4 × 5	5RM								
Forward box step-up	73	3 × 12	3 × 12	3 × 12	2 × 12								
Standing two-way calf raise	77	3 × 12	3 × 12	3 × 12	2 × 12					3 × 12	3 × 12	3 × 12	2 × 12
Pull-up	33	1 × 6	2 × 6	2 × 6	1 × 6								
Push press	130					4 × 6	4 × 6	4 × 6	2 × 6				
Front squat	66					4 × 8	4 × 6	4 × 5	5RM				
Romanian deadlift	67					4 × 8	4 × 8	4 × 8	2 × 8				
Dumbbell rotator cuff routine	44					5 × 10	5 × 10	5 × 12	5 × 12				
Lat pull-down	56					3 × 8	3 × 8	3 × 8					
Glute–ham: straight leg	71					3 × 12	3 × 12	3 × 15	2 × 12				
Power clean	129									3 × 6	4 × 5	4 × 5	5RM
Bench press (incline)	55									3 × 8	4 × 8	4 × 8	6RM
Seated row	57									4 × 8	4 × 8	4 × 8	2 × 8
Glute–ham: bent knee	92									3 × 10	3 × 10	3 × 10	2 × 10
General abs	169	Prog A	Prog A	Prog A	Prog A					Prog A	Prog A	Prog A	Prog A
Advanced abs	169					Prog B	Prog B	Prog B	Prog B				
Low-intensity plyometrics	133	1-2 sets	2 sets	2 sets	1 set					1-2 sets	2 sets	2 sets	1 set

SPRINTS

199

Off-Season 12-Week Program—Weeks 9 Through 12

Exercise	Page #	Monday				Wednesday				Friday			
		1	2	3	4	1	2	3	4	1	2	3	4
Power shrug	125	3 × 4	3 × 4	3 × 3	3 × 3								
Power clean	129	4 × 4	5 × 4	5 × 3	3RM								
Back squat	65	4 × 6	5 × 5	4 × 4	3RM								
Shoulder press (standing)	55	4 × 6	4 × 5	4 × 4	3 × 4								
Lat pull-down	56	3 × 8	3 × 8	3 × 8	2 × 8								
Standing two-way calf raise	77	2 × 15	2 × 15	2 × 15	2 × 15					3 × 10	3 × 10	3 × 10	2 × 10
Hang clean	127					4 × 4	4 × 3	4 × 3	3RM				
Traditional deadlift	68					4 × 6	4 × 6	4 × 6	2 × 6				
Bench press	55					4 × 5	4 × 4	4 × 3	3RM				
Seated row	57					4 × 8	4 × 8	4 × 8	2 × 8				
Glute–ham: straight leg	71					3 × 12	3 × 12	3 × 15	2 × 12				
Dumbbell rotator cuff routine	44					5 × 15	5 × 15	5 × 15	5 × 15				
Power clean	129									4 × 5	5 × 4	5 × 3	3 × 3
Front squat	66									4 × 6	4 × 5	4 × 5	5RM
Bench press (incline)	55									4 × 8	4 × 6	4 × 5	2 × 5
Glute–ham: bent knee	92									3 × 10	3 × 10	3 × 10	2 × 10
General abs	169	Prog A	Prog A	Prog A	Prog A					Prog A	Prog A	Prog A	Prog A
Advanced abs	169					Prog B	Prog B	Prog B	Prog B				
Low-intensity plyometrics	133									1-2 sets	2 sets	2 sets	1 set
Moderate-intensity plyometrics	136	1-2 sets	2 sets	2 sets	1 set								

Preseason 8-Week Program—Weeks 1 Through 4

Exercise	Page #	Monday 1	2	3	4	Wednesday 1	2	3	4	Friday 1	2	3	4
Power shrug	125	3 × 4	3 × 4	3 × 3	3 × 3								
Power clean	129	4 × 4	5 × 3	5 × 3	2 × 3								
Front squat	66	4 × 8	4 × 6	4 × 4	2 × 4								
Bench press (incline)	55	3 × 6	3 × 5	3 × 4	2 × 4								
Lat pull-down	56	3 × 8	3 × 8	3 × 8	2 × 8								
Dumbbell rotator cuff routine	44	5 × 15	5 × 15	5 × 15	5 × 15					5 × 15	5 × 15	5 × 15	5 × 15
Hang clean	127					4 × 4	4 × 3	4 × 3	3 × 3				
Traditional deadlift	68					4 × 6	4 × 6	4 × 6	2 × 6				
Bench press	55					3 × 6	3 × 6	3 × 5	3 × 4				
Glute–ham: bent knee	92					4 × 8	4 × 10	4 × 10	2 × 10				
Standing two-way calf raise	77					3 × 12	3 × 12	3 × 15	2 × 12				
Power clean	129									4 × 4	5 × 3	5 × 3	2 × 3
Back squat	65									4 × 6	4 × 5	4 × 5	3 × 5
Push press	130									4 × 4	4 × 4	4 × 4	3 × 4
Seated row	57									4 × 8	4 × 6	4 × 6	2 × 6
Shoulder press (standing)	55									3 × 10	3 × 10	3 × 10	2 × 10
General abs	169									Prog A	Prog A	Prog A	Prog A
Advanced abs	169					Prog B	Prog B	Prog B	Prog B				
High-intensity plyometrics	141									1-2 sest	2 sets	2 sets	1 set
Agility drills	118	1-2 sets	2 sets	2 sets	1 set								

Preseason 8-Week Program—Weeks 5 Through 8

Exercise	Page #	Monday 1	Monday 2	Monday 3	Monday 4	Wednesday 1	Wednesday 2	Wednesday 3	Wednesday 4	Friday 1	Friday 2	Friday 3	Friday 4
Power shrug	125	3 × 3	3 × 3	3 × 3	3 × 3								
Power clean	129	5 × 3	5 × 2	4 × 2	1RM					4 × 4	5 × 3	5 × 3	3 × 3
Back squat	65	5 × 3	5 × 3	4 × 2	1RM					4 × 6	4 × 5	4 × 5	3 × 5
Bench press (incline)	55	4 × 5	4 × 4	4 × 3	3RM								
Forward box step-up	73	3 × 12	3 × 12	3 × 12									
Standing two-way calf raise	77	3 × 12	3 × 12	3 × 12		3 × 12	3 × 12	3 × 12					
Hang clean	127					4 × 3	4 × 3	4 × 2	1RM				
Front squat	66					5 × 4	5 × 3	4 × 2	1RM				
Bench press	55					5 × 3	5 × 3	4 × 2	1RM				
Glute–ham: bent knee	92					3 × 12	3 × 12	3 × 12					
Dumbbell rotator cuff routine	44					5 × 15	5 × 15	5 × 15	5 × 15	5 × 15	5 × 15	5 × 15	5 × 15
Shoulder press (standing)	55									4 × 4	4 × 4	4 × 4	3 × 4
Lat pull-down	56									4 × 4	4 × 4	4 × 4	3 × 4
General abs	169									Prog A	Prog A	Prog A	Prog A
Advanced abs	169					Prog B	Prog B	Prog B	Prog B				
High-intensity plyometrics	141									1-2 sets	2 sets	2 sets	1 set
Agility drills	118	1-2 sets	2 ets	2 sets	1 set								

In-Season Maintenance 4-Week Program—Weeks 1 Through 4

Exercise	Page #	Monday				Wednesday			
		1	2	3	4	1	2	3	4
Power clean	129	3 × 3	3 × 3	3 × 2	3 × 3				
Back squat	65	3 × 4	3 × 4	3 × 3	2 × 4				
Bench press (incline)	55	3 × 6	3 × 5	3 × 4	3 × 3				
Forward box step-up	73	3 × 10	3 × 12	3 × 12					
Hang clean	127					3 × 3	3 × 3	3 × 2	3 × 2
Front squat	66					3 × 6	3 × 5	3 × 4	3 × 3
Bench press	55					3 × 4	3 × 4	3 × 3	3 × 3
Glute–ham: bent knee	92					3 × 12	3 × 12	3 × 12	3 × 8
Seated row	57					3 × 8	3 × 8	3 × 8	
Advanced abs	169					Prog B	Prog B	Prog B	Prog B
Moderate-intensity plyometrics	136	1-2 sets	2 sets	2 sets	1 set				

SWIMMING

Off-Season 12-Week Program—Weeks 1 Through 4

Exercise	Page #	Monday 1	2	3	4	Wednesday 1	2	3	4	Friday 1	2	3	4
Back squat	65	3 × 8	3 × 10	3 × 10	2 × 10								
Bench press (dumbbell)	55	3 × 8	3 × 10	3 × 12	2 × 10								
Lat pull-down	56	3 × 8	3 × 10	3 × 12	2 × 10					3 × 8	3 × 10	3 × 12	3 × 12
Glute–ham: bent knee	92	2 × 8	2 × 10	2 × 10	2 × 8								
Glute–ham: straight leg	71	2 × 10	2 × 10	2 × 12	2 × 8					2 × 10	2 × 10	2 × 12	2 × 12
Walking lunge	72					3 × 8	3 × 10	3 × 10	2 × 8				
Shoulder press (dumbbell)	55					3 × 8	3 × 10	3 × 12	2 × 8				
Hip hike	99					3 × 8	3 × 10	3 × 10	2 × 8				
Seated row	57					2 × 8	2 × 10	2 × 12	2 × 8				
Lateral raise	47					2 × 8	2 × 10	2 × 10	2 × 8				
Front squat	66									3 × 8	3 × 10	3 × 12	3 × 15
Bridge push-up	97									3 × 12	3 × 12	3 × 15	3 × 15
Single-leg hamstring curl	70									2 × 8	2 × 10	2 × 10	2 × 12
General abs	169	Prog A	Prog A	Prog A	Prog A	Prog A	Prog A	Prog A	Prog A	Prog A	Prog A	Prog A	Prog A

Hold each flexibility exercise for a count of 8 to 10.

Off-Season 12-Week Program—Weeks 5 Through 8

Exercise	Page #	Monday 1	Monday 2	Monday 3	Monday 4	Wednesday 1	Wednesday 2	Wednesday 3	Wednesday 4	Friday 1	Friday 2	Friday 3	Friday 4
Push press	130	3 × 6	3 × 6	3 × 5	2 × 5					3 × 6	3 × 5	3 × 4	2 × 4
Front squat	66	3 × 8	3 × 10	3 × 10	2 × 8								
Lat pull-down	56	2 × 10	2 × 10	2 × 8	2 × 8								
Shoulder press	55	3 × 10	3 × 10	3 × 10	2 × 8								
Single-leg hamstring curl	70	3 × 8	3 × 10	3 × 12	2 × 8								
Glute–ham: straight leg	71	2 × 10	2 × 12	2 × 12	2 × 10								
Hang clean	127					3 × 6	3 × 6	3 × 5	2 × 5				
Back squat	65					3 × 8	3 × 6	3 × 8	2 × 8				
Forward box step-up	73					2 × 12	2 × 12	2 × 12	2 × 10				
Bench press (incline, dumbbell)	55					3 × 10	3 × 8	3 × 8	2 × 8				
Seated row	57					3 × 10	3 × 10	3 × 10	2 × 10	2 × 10	2 × 10	2 × 12	2 × 10
Front or lateral raise	46 or 47					2 × 10	2 × 10	2 × 10	2 × 8				
Romanian deadlift	67									3 × 8	3 × 8	3 × 8	2 × 8
Bridge push-up	97									3 × 12	3 × 15	3 × 15	2 × 10
Single-leg knee extension	70									3 × 8	3 × 10	3 × 12	2 × 8
Standing two-way calf raise	77									2 × 10	2 × 12	2 × 12	2 × 10
General abs	169	Prog A	Prog A	Prog A	Prog A	Prog A	Prog A	Prog A	Prog A	Prog A	Prog A	Prog A	Prog A

Hold each flexibility exercise for a count of 8 to 10.

Off-Season 12-Week Program—Weeks 9 Through 12

Exercise	Page #	Monday 1	2	3	4	Wednesday 1	2	3	4	Friday 1	2	3	4
Push press	130	3 × 5	3 × 4	3 × 4	2 × 4								
Front squat	66	3 × 4	3 × 6	3 × 6	2 × 6								
Lat pull-down	56	2 × 10	2 × 10	2 × 8	2 × 8								
Shoulder press	55	3 × 8	3 × 8	3 × 8	2 × 8								
Walking lunge	72	3 × 8	3 × 8	3 × 8	2 × 8								
Glute–ham: straight leg	71	2 × 12	2 × 14	2 × 14	2 × 12								
Hang clean	127					3 × 5	3 × 5	3 × 4	2 × 4				
Back squat	65					3 × 8	3 × 6	3 × 6	2 × 6				
Forward box step-up	73					2 × 6	2 × 6	2 × 6	2 × 6				
Bench press (incline, dumbbell)	55					3 × 8	3 × 6	3 × 6	2 × 6				
Seated row	57					3 × 8	3 × 8	3 × 8	2 × 8	2 × 8	2 × 8	2 × 8	2 × 8
Front or lateral raise	46 or 47					2 × 10	2 × 10	2 × 10	2 × 8				
Romanian deadlift	67									3 × 8	3 × 8	3 × 8	2 × 8
Bridge push-up	97									3 × 12	3 × 15	3 × 5	2 × 10
Single-leg knee extension	70									3 × 10	3 × 10	3 × 10	2 × 8
Standing two-way calf raise	77									2 × 12	2 × 15	2 × 15	2 × 10
General abs	169	Prog A	Prog A	Prog A	Prog A	Prog A	Prog A	Prog A	Prog A	Prog A	Prog A	Prog A	Prog A

Hold each flexibility exercise for a count of 8 to 10.

Preseason 8-Week Program—Weeks 1 Through 4

Exercise	Page #	Monday 1	Monday 2	Monday 3	Monday 4	Wednesday 1	Wednesday 2	Wednesday 3	Wednesday 4	Friday 1	Friday 2	Friday 3	Friday 4
Power clean	129	3 × 4	3 × 4	3 × 3	3 × 3								
Front squat	66	3 × 6	3 × 6	3 × 6	2 × 6								
Lat pull-down	56	2 × 8	2 × 8	2 × 8	2 × 8								
Glute–ham: bent knee	92	3 × 8	3 × 8	3 × 8	2 × 8								
Forearm push-up	52	3 × 8	3 × 8	3 × 8	2 × 8								
Glute–ham: straight leg	71	2 × 12	2 × 14	2 × 14	2 × 12								
Hang clean	127					3 × 5	3 × 5	3 × 4	2 × 4				
Back squat	65					3 × 6	3 × 6	3 × 6	2 × 6				
Forward box step-up	73					2 × 6	2 × 6	2 × 6	2 × 6				
Bench press (incline, dumbbell)	55					3 × 8	3 × 6	3 × 6	2 × 6				
Seated row	57					3 × 8	3 × 8	3 × 8	2 × 8	2 × 8	2 × 8	2 × 8	2 × 8
Front or lateral raise	46 or 47					2 × 10	2 × 10	2 × 10	2 × 8				
Romanian deadlift	67									3 × 8	3 × 8	3 × 8	2 × 8
Bridge push-up	97									3 × 12	3 × 15	3 × 15	2 × 10
Standing two-way calf raise	77									3 × 10	3 × 10	3 × 10	2 × 8
General abs	169	Prog A	Prog A	Prog A	Prog A	Prog A	Prog A	Prog A	Prog A	Prog A	Prog A	Prog A	Prog A

Hold each flexibility exercise for a count of 8 to 10.

SWIMMING

Preseason 8-Week Program—Weeks 5 Through 8

Exercise	Page #	Monday 1	Monday 2	Monday 3	Monday 4	Wednesday 1	Wednesday 2	Wednesday 3	Wednesday 4	Friday 1	Friday 2	Friday 3	Friday 4
Power clean	129	3 × 4	3 × 4	3 × 3	3 × 3								
Push press	130	3 × 4	3 × 4	3 × 3	3 × 3								
Back squat	65	3 × 6	3 × 6	3 × 6	2 × 6								
Lat pull-down	56	2 × 8	2 × 8	2 × 8	2 × 8								
Glute–ham: straight leg	71	3 × 8	3 × 8	3 × 8	2 × 8								
Hang clean	127					3 × 4	3 × 4	3 × 3	3 × 2				
Front squat	66					3 × 4	3 × 4	3 × 3	3 × 2				
Bench press (incline, dumbbell)	55					3 × 8	3 × 6	3 × 6	2 × 6				
Forward box step-up	73					2 × 6	2 × 6	2 × 6	2 × 6				
Seated row	57					3 × 8	3 × 8	3 × 8	2 × 8	2 × 8	2 × 8	2 × 8	2 × 8
Romanian deadlift	67									3 × 8	3 × 8	3 × 8	2 × 8
Bridge push-up	97									3 × 12	3 × 15	3 × 15	2 × 10
Standing two-way calf raise	77									2 × 12	2 × 15	2 × 15	2 × 10
General abs	169	Prog A	Prog A	Prog A	Prog A	Prog A	Prog A	Prog A	Prog A	Prog A	Prog A	Prog A	Prog A

Hold each flexibility exercise for a count of 8 to 10.

In-Season Maintenance 4-Week Program—Weeks 1 Through 4

Exercise	Page #	Monday				Wednesday			
		1	2	3	4	1	2	3	4
Power clean	129	3 × 4	3 × 4	3 × 3	3 × 3				
Front squat	66	3 × 6	3 × 5	3 × 6	2 × 5				
Romanian deadlift	67	2 × 8	2 × 8	2 × 8	2 × 8				
Seated row	57	3 × 8	3 × 8	3 × 8	2 × 8				
Hang clean	127					3 × 4	3 × 4	3 × 3	2 × 3
Push press	130					3 × 4	3 × 4	3 × 3	2 × 3
Forward box step-up	73					2 × 6	2 × 6	2 × 6	2 × 6
Lat pull-down	56					3 × 8	3 × 8	3 × 8	2 × 8
General abs	169	Prog A	Prog A	Prog A	Prog A	Prog A	Prog A	Prog A	Prog A

Hold each flexibility exercise for a count of 8 to 10.

THROWING

Off-Season 12-Week Program—Weeks 1 Through 4

Exercise	Page #	Monday 1	Monday 2	Monday 3	Monday 4	Wednesday 1	Wednesday 2	Wednesday 3	Wednesday 4	Friday 1	Friday 2	Friday 3	Friday 4
Back squat	65	4 × 12	4 × 10	4 × 8	3 × 8								
Shoulder press (standing)	55	4 × 12	4 × 10	4 × 10	2 × 10								
Walking lunge	72	3 × 12	3 × 12	3 × 12	2 × 12								
Forward box step-up	73	4 × 12	4 × 12	4 × 12	2 × 12								
Lat pull-down	56	3 × 12	3 × 10	3 × 10	2 × 10								
Traditional deadlift	68					4 × 12	4 × 10	4 × 8	3 × 8				
Push press	130					4 × 10	4 × 8	4 × 6	3 × 6				
Single-leg knee extension	70					4 × 12	4 × 12	4 × 10	2 × 10				
Glute–ham: straight leg	71					3 × 10	3 × 12	3 × 15	2 × 15				
Seated row	57					3 × 12	3 × 12	3 × 10	3 × 8	4 × 12	4 × 10	4 × 8	3 × 8
Front squat	66									4 × 10	4 × 10	4 × 10	2 × 10
Romanian deadlift	67									3 × 10	3 × 10	4 × 10	2 × 10
Bench press	55									4 × 12	4 × 10	4 × 8	3 × 8
Shoulder press (seated)	55									4 × 12	4 × 10	4 × 8	3 × 8
General abs	169	Prog A	Prog A	Prog A	Prog A					Prog A	Prog A	Prog A	Prog A
Advanced abs	169	Prog B	Prog B	Prog B	Prog B					Prog B	Prog B	Prog B	Prog B
Jump rope drills	124					1 set	1-2 sets	2 sets	2 sets				

Off-Season 12-Week Program—Weeks 5 Through 8

Exercise	Page #	Monday 1	2	3	4	Wednesday 1	2	3	4	Friday 1	2	3	4
Power shrug	125	3 × 4	3 × 4	3 × 3	3 × 3								
Hang clean	126	4 × 6	4 × 6	4 × 5	5RM	4 × 4	4 × 4	4 × 3	3RM				
High pull	127	3 × 3	3 × 3	3 × 3						3 × 3	3 × 3	3 × 3	3 × 3
Back squat	65	4 × 8	4 × 6	4 × 5	5RM								
Shoulder press (standing)	55	4 × 8	4 × 6	4 × 5	5RM								
Pull-up	33	1 × 10	2 × 10	2 × 10	1 × 10								
Push press	130					4 × 6	4 × 6	4 × 6	2 × 6				
Front squat	66					4 × 8	4 × 6	4 × 5	5RM				
Romanian deadlift	67					4 × 8	4 × 8	4 × 8	2 × 8				
Seated row	57					3 × 10	3 × 10	3 × 10	2 × 10	4 × 8	4 × 8	4 × 8	2 × 8
Glute–ham: straight leg	71					3 × 12	3 × 12	3 × 15	2 × 12				
Power clean	129									3 × 6	4 × 5	4 × 5	5RM
Bench press (incline)	55									3 × 8	4 × 8	4 × 8	6RM
Glute–ham: bent knee	92									3 × 10	3 × 10	3 × 10	2 × 10
Forward box step-up	73									3 × 12	3 × 12	3 × 12	2 × 12
General abs	169	Prog A	Prog A	Prog A	Prog A					Prog A	Prog A	Prog A	Prog A
Advanced abs	169					Prog B	Prog B	Prog B	Prog B				
Low-intensity plyometrics	133	1-2 sets	2 sets	2 sets	1 set					1-2 sets	2 sets	2 sets	1 set

THROWING

Off-Season 12-Week Program—Weeks 9 Through 12

Exercise	Page #	Monday 1	Monday 2	Monday 3	Monday 4	Wednesday 1	Wednesday 2	Wednesday 3	Wednesday 4	Friday 1	Friday 2	Friday 3	Friday 4
Power shrug	125	3 × 4	3 × 4	3 × 3	3 × 3								
Power clean	129	4 × 4	5 × 4	5 × 3	3RM					4 × 5	5 × 4	5 × 3	3 × 3
Back squat	65	4 × 6	5 × 5	4 × 4	3RM								
Shoulder press (standing)	55	4 × 6	4 × 5	4 × 4	3 × 4								
Lat pull-down	56	3 × 8	3 × 8	3 × 8	2 × 8								
Hang clean followed by push press	127 & 130					4 × 4	4 × 3	4 × 3	3 × 3				
Traditional deadlift	68					4 × 6	4 × 6	4 × 6	2 × 6				
Bench press	55					4 × 5	4 × 4	4 × 3	3RM				
Seated row	57					4 × 8	4 × 8	4 × 8	2 × 8				
Glute–ham: straight leg	71					3 × 12	3 × 12	3 × 15	2 × 12				
Front squat	66									4 × 6	4 × 5	4 × 5	5RM
Push press	130									4 × 6	4 × 5	4 × 5	3 × 4
Bench press (incline)	55									4 × 8	4 × 6	4 × 5	2 × 5
Glute–ham: bent knee	92									3 × 10	3 × 10	3 × 10	2 × 10
General abs	169	Prog A	Prog A	Prog A	Prog A					1-2 sets	2 sets	2 sets	1 set
Advanced abs	169					Prog B	Prog B	Prog B	Prog B				
Low-intensity plyometrics	133									1-2 sets	2 sets	2 sets	1 set
Moderate-intensity plyometrics	136	1-2 sets	2 sets	2 sets	1 set								

Preseason 8-Week Program—Weeks 1 Through 4

Exercise	Page #	Monday 1	Monday 2	Monday 3	Monday 4	Wednesday 1	Wednesday 2	Wednesday 3	Wednesday 4	Friday 1	Friday 2	Friday 3	Friday 4
Power shrug	125	3 × 4	3 × 4	3 × 3	3 × 3								
Power clean	129	4 × 4	5 × 3	5 × 3	2 × 3								
Front squat	66	4 × 8	4 × 6	4 × 4	2 × 4								
Bench press (incline)	55	4 × 6	4 × 5	4 × 4	3 × 4								
Lat pull-down	56	3 × 8	3 × 8	3 × 8	2 × 8								
Hang clean	127					4 × 4	4 × 3	4 × 3	3 × 3				
Traditional deadlift	68					4 × 6	4 × 6	4 × 6	2 × 6				
Bench press	55					4 × 6	4 × 6	4 × 5	3 × 4				
Glute–ham: bent knee	92					4 × 8	4 × 10	4 × 10	2 × 10				
Glute–ham: straight leg	71					3 × 12	3 × 12	3 × 15	2 × 12				
Power clean	129									4 × 4	5 × 3	5 × 3	2 × 3
Back squat	65									4 × 6	4 × 5	4 × 5	3 × 5
Push press	130									4 × 4	4 × 4	4 × 4	3 × 4
Seated row	57									4 × 8	4 × 6	4 × 6	2 × 6
Dumbbell rotator cuff routine (5 lb or 2 kg)	44									3 × 10	3 × 10	3 × 10	2 × 10
General abs	169									Prog A	Prog A	Prog A	Prog A
Advanced abs	169					Prog B	Prog B	Prog B	Prog B				
High-intensity plyometrics	141									1-2 sest	2 sets	2 sets	1 set
Agility drills	118	1-2 sets	2 sets	2 sets	1 set								

213

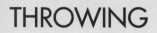

THROWING

Preseason 8-Week Program—Weeks 5 Through 8

Exercise	Page #	Monday 1	Monday 2	Monday 3	Monday 4	Wednesday 1	Wednesday 2	Wednesday 3	Wednesday 4	Friday 1	Friday 2	Friday 3	Friday 4
Power shrug	125	3 × 3	3 × 3	3 × 3	3 × 3								
Power clean	129	5 × 3	5 × 2	4 × 2	1RM								
Back squat	65	5 × 3	5 × 3	4 × 2	1RM					4 × 5	4 × 5	4 × 5	3 × 5
Bench press (incline)	55	3 × 5	3 × 4	3 × 4	3RM								
Forward box step-up	73	3 × 12	3 × 12	3 × 12									
Hang clean	127					4 × 3	4 × 3	4 × 2	1RM				
Front squat	66					5 × 4	5 × 3	4 × 2	1RM				
Bench press	55					3 × 3	3 × 3	3 × 2	1RM				
Glute–ham: bent knee	92					3 × 12	3 × 12	3 × 12					
Glute–ham: straight leg	71					3 × 12	3 × 12	3 × 15					
Push press	130									4 × 4	5 × 3	5 × 3	3 × 3
Shoulder press (standing)	55									4 × 4	4 × 4	4 × 4	3 × 4
Lat pull-down	56									4 × 8	3 × 8	3 × 8	3 × 8
Dumbbell rotator cuff routine (5 lb or 2 kg)	44									3 × 10	3 × 10	3 × 10	3 × 10
General abs	169									Prog A	Prog A	Prog A	Prog A
Advanced abs	169					Prog B	Prog B	Prog B	Prog B				
High-intensity plyometrics	141	1-2 sets	2 sets	2 sets	1 set	1-2 sets	2 sets	2 sets	1 set	1-2 sets	2 sets	2 sets	1 set
Agility drills	118	1-2 sets	2 sets	2 sets	1 set								

In-Season Maintenance 4-Week Program—Weeks 1 Through 4

Exercise	Page #	Monday 1	2	3	4	Wednesday 1	2	3	4
Power shrug	125	3 × 3	3 × 3	3 × 3	3 × 3				
Power clean	129	4 × 3	4 × 3	4 × 2	3 × 3				
Back squat	65	3 × 5	3 × 4	3 × 3	2 × 4				
Bench press (incline)	55	3 × 6	3 × 5	3 × 4	3 × 3				
Forward box step-ups	73	3 × 10	3 × 12	3 × 12					
Hang clean	127					3 × 3	3 × 3	3 × 2	3 × 2
Front squat	66					3 × 6	3 × 5	3 × 4	3 × 3
Bench press	55					3 × 4	3 × 4	3 × 3	3 × 3
Glute–ham: bent knee	92					3 × 12	3 × 12	3 × 12	3 × 8
Glute–ham: straight leg	71					3 × 12	3 × 12	3 × 15	
Advanced abs	169					Prog B	Prog B	Prog B	Prog B
Moderate-intensity plyometrics	136	1-2 sets	2 sets	2 sets	1 set				

TRIATHLON

Off-Season 12-Week Program

Exercise	Page #	Weeks 1-4			Weeks 5-8			Weeks 9-12		
		Day 1	Day 2	Day 3	Day 1	Day 2	Day 3	Day 1	Day 2	Day 3
General strength										
Walking lunge	72	4 × 15		4 × 15	4 × 15		4 × 15	4 × 15		4 × 15
Bench press (incline)	55	3 × 12		3 × 12	3 × 10		3 × 10	3 × 8		3 × 8
Single-leg knee extension	70	3 × 12		3 × 12	3 × 10		3 × 10	3 × 8		3 × 8
Lat pull-down	56	3 × 12		3 × 12	3 × 10		3 × 10	3 × 8		3 × 8
Leg curl	103	3 × 12		3 × 12	3 × 10		3 × 10	3 × 8		3 × 8
Seated row	54	3 × 12		3 × 12	3 × 10		3 × 10	3 × 8		3 × 8
Dumbbell rotator cuff routine (5 lb or 2 kg)	44	5 × 10		5 × 10	5 × 12		5 × 12	5 × 15		5 × 15
Glute–ham: straight leg	71	1 × 15		1 × 15	2 × 15		2 × 15	2 × 15		2 × 15
Glute–ham: bent knee	92	1 × 15		1 × 15	1 × 15		1 × 15	2 × 15		2 × 15
General abs	169	Prog A		Prog A	Prog A		Prog A	Prog A		Prog A
Power										
Split jump	137		3 × 10			3 × 10			3 × 10	
Power push-up	55		3 × 6			3 × 8			3 × 10	
High pull	126		3 × 6			3 × 5			3 × 5	
Shuffle squat	77		2 × 10			2 × 15			2 × 15	
Medicine ball: overhead throw	95		2 × 15			2 × 15			2 × 15	
Medicine ball: chest pass	93		2 × 15			2 × 15			2 × 15	
Physioball swimmer	58		2 × 15			2 × 15			2 × 15	
Extended crunch with pass	104		3 × 10			3 × 10			3 × 10	

Choose two of the three leg exercises on day 1 and day 3 (for example, leg extension and walking lunge).

Preseason 4-Week Program

Exercise	Page #	Weeks 1-2			Weeks 3-4		
		Day 1	Day 2	Day 3	Day 1	Day 2	Day 3
General strength							
Walking lunge	72	3 × 15		2 × 15	3 × 15		2 × 15
Bench press (incline)	55	3 × 8		2 × 8	2 × 10		2 × 8
Single-leg knee extension	70	3 × 8		2 × 8	2 × 10		2 × 8
Lat pull-down	56	3 × 8		2 × 8	2 × 10		2 × 8
Leg curl	103	3 × 8		2 × 8	2 × 10		2 × 8
Seated row	57	3 × 8		2 × 8	3 × 8		2 × 8
Dumbbell rotator cuff routine (5 lb or 2 kg)	44	5 × 10		5 × 10	5 × 12		5 × 10
Glute–ham: straight leg	71	1 × 15		1 × 15	2 × 15		2 × 15
Glute–ham: bent knee	92	1 × 15		1 × 15	1 × 15		1 × 15
General abs	169	Prog A		Prog A	Prog A		Prog A
Power							
Split jump	137		3 × 10	O		3 × 10	O
Shuffle squat	75		3 × 6	P		3 × 8	P
High pull	126		3 × 6	T		3 × 5	T
Side lunge	75		2 × 10	I		2 × 15	I
Medicine ball: overhead throw	95		2 × 15	O		2 × 15	O
Medicine ball: chest pass	93		2 × 15	N		2 × 15	N
Physioball swimmer	58		2 × 15	A		2 × 15	A
Extended crunch with pass	104		2 × 15	L		2 × 15	L

In-Season Maintenance 16-Week Program

Exercise	Page #	Weeks 1-16		
		Day 1	Day 2	Day 3
General strength				
Walking lunge	72	2 × 15		2 × 15
Bench press (incline)	55	2 × 12	O	2 × 10
Single-leg knee extension	70	2 × 12	P	2 × 10
Lat pull-down	56	2 × 12	T	2 × 10
Leg curl	103	2 × 12	I	2 × 10
Seated row	57	2 × 12	O	2 × 10
Dumbbell rotator cuff routine (5 lb or 2 kg)	44	5 × 15	N	5 × 15
Glute–ham: straight leg	71	1 × 15	A	1 × 15
Glute–ham: bent knee	92	1 × 15	L	1 × 15
General abs	169	Prog A		
Power				
Split jump	137		2 × 10	
Power push-up	56		2 × 8	
High pull	126		2 × 6	
Side lunge	75		2 × 10	
Medicine ball: overhead throw	95		2 × 15	
Medicine ball: chest pass	93		2 × 15	
Physioball swimmer	58		2 × 15	
Extended crunch with pass	104		2 × 15	

Off-Season 12-Week Program—Weeks 1 Through 4

Exercise	Page #	Monday				Wednesday				Friday			
		1	2	3	4	1	2	3	4	1	2	3	4
Back squat	65	4 × 12	4 × 10	4 × 8	3 × 8								
Shoulder press (standing)	55	4 × 12	4 × 10	4 × 10	2 × 10					4 × 12	4 × 10	4 × 8	3 × 8
Walking lunge	72	3 × 12	3 × 12	3 × 12	2 × 12								
Forward box step-up	73	4 × 12	4 × 12	4 × 12	2 × 12								
Lat pull-down	56	3 × 12	3 × 12	3 × 12	2 × 12								
Standing two-way calf raise	77												
Traditional deadlift	68					4 × 12	4 × 10	4 × 8	3 × 8				
Push press	130					4 × 10	4 × 8	4 × 6	3 × 6				
Single-leg knee extension	70					4 × 12	4 × 12	4 × 10	2 × 10				
Glute–ham: straight leg	71					3 × 10	3 × 12	3 × 15	2 × 15				
Seated row	57					3 × 12	3 × 12	3 × 10	3 × 8	4 × 12	4 × 10	4 × 8	3 × 8
Front squat	66									4 × 10	4 × 10	4 × 10	2 × 10
Romanian deadlift	67									3 × 10	3 × 10	4 × 10	2 × 10
Bench press	55									4 × 12	4 × 10	4 × 8	3 × 8
General abs	169	Prog A	Prog A	Prog A	Prog A					Prog A	Prog A	Prog A	Prog A
Advanced abs	169	Prog B	Prog B	Prog B	Prog B					Prog B	Prog B	Prog B	Prog B
Jump rope drills	124					1 set	1-2 sets	2 sets	2 sets				

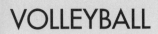

VOLLEYBALL

Off-Season 12-Week Program—Weeks 5 Through 8

Exercise	Page #	Monday 1	2	3	4	Wednesday 1	2	3	4	Friday 1	2	3	4
Power shrug	125	3 × 4	3 × 4	3 × 3	3 × 3								
Hang clean	127	4 × 6	4 × 6	4 × 5	5RM	4 × 4	4 × 4	4 × 3	3 × 6	3 × 3	3 × 3	3 × 3	3 × 3
High pull	126	3 × 3	3 × 3	3 × 3									
Back squat	65	4 × 8	4 × 6	4 × 5	5RM								
Forward box step-up	73	3 × 12	3 × 12	3 × 12	2 × 12								
Standing two-way calf raise	77	3 × 12	3 × 12	3 × 12	2 × 12					3 × 12	3 × 12	3 × 12	2 × 12
Pull-up	33	1 × 10	2 × 10	2 × 10	1 × 10								
Push press	130					4 × 6	4 × 6	4 × 6	2 × 6				
Front squat	66					4 × 8	4 × 6	4 × 5	5RM				
Romanian deadlift	67					4 × 8	4 × 8	4 × 8	2 × 8				
Dumbbell rotator cuff routine	44					5 × 6	5 × 6	5 × 6	5 × 6				
Three-way weight transfer	76					3 × 8	3 × 8	3 × 8					
Glute–ham: straight leg	71					3 × 12	3 × 12	3 × 15	2 × 12				
Power clean	129									3 × 5	4 × 5	4 × 5	5RM
Bench press (incline)	55									3 × 8	4 × 8	4 × 8	6RM
Seated row	57									4 × 8	4 × 8	4 × 8	2 × 8
Glute–ham: bent knee	92									3 × 10	3 × 10	3 × 10	2 × 10
General abs	169	Prog A	Prog A	Prog A	Prog A					Prog A	Prog A	Prog A	Prog A
Advanced abs	169					Prog B	Prog B	Prog B	Prog B				
Low-intensity plyometrics	133	1-2 sets	2 sets	2 sets	1 set					1-2 sets	2 sets	2 sets	1 set

Off-Season 12-Week Program—Weeks 9 Through 12

Exercise	Page #	Monday 1	Monday 2	Monday 3	Monday 4	Wednesday 1	Wednesday 2	Wednesday 3	Wednesday 4	Friday 1	Friday 2	Friday 3	Friday 4
Power shrug	125	3 × 4	3 × 4	3 × 3	3 × 3								
Power clean	129	4 × 4	5 × 4	5 × 3	3RM					4 × 5	5 × 4	5 × 3	3 × 3
Back squat	65	4 × 6	5 × 5	4 × 4	3RM								
Shoulder press (standing)	55	4 × 6	4 × 5	4 × 4	3 × 4								
Lat pull-down	56	3 × 8	3 × 8	3 × 8	2 × 8								
Dumbbell rotator cuff routine	44	5 × 8	5 × 8	5 × 8	5 × 8					5 × 8	5 × 8	5 × 8	5 × 8
Hang clean	127					4 × 4	4 × 4	4 × 3	3RM				
Romanian deadlift	67					4 × 6	4 × 6	4 × 6	2 × 6				
Bench press	55					4 × 5	4 × 4	4 × 3	3RM				
Seated row	57					4 × 8	4 × 8	4 × 8	2 × 8				
Glute–ham: straight leg	71					3 × 12	3 × 12	3 × 15	2 × 12				
Standing two-way calf raise	77					2 × 15	2 × 15	2 × 15	2 × 15	3 × 10	3 × 10	3 × 10	2 × 10
Front squat	66									4 × 6	4 × 5	4 × 5	5RM
Bench press (incline)	55									4 × 8	4 × 6	4 × 5	2 × 5
Glute–ham: bent knee	92									3 × 10	3 × 10	3 × 10	2 × 10
General abs	169	Prog A	Prog A	Prog A	Prog A					Prog A	Prog A	Prog A	Prog A
Advanced abs	169					Prog B	Prog B	Prog B	Prog B				
Low-intensity plyometrics	133									1-2 sets	2 sets	2 sets	1 set
Moderate-intensity plyometrics	136	1-2 sets	2 sets	2 sets	1 set								

VOLLEYBALL

Preseason 8-Week Program—Weeks 1 Through 4

Exercise	Page #	Monday 1	Monday 2	Monday 3	Monday 4	Wednesday 1	Wednesday 2	Wednesday 3	Wednesday 4	Friday 1	Friday 2	Friday 3	Friday 4
Power shrug	125	3 × 4	3 × 4	3 × 3	3 × 3								
Power clean	129	4 × 4	5 × 3	5 × 3	2 × 3					4 × 4	5 × 3	5 × 3	2 × 3
Front squat	66	4 × 8	4 × 6	4 × 4	2 × 4								
Bench press (incline)	55	3 × 6	3 × 5	3 × 4	2 × 4								
Lat pull-down	56	3 × 8	3 × 8	3 × 8	2 × 8								
Dumbbell rotator cuff routine	44	5 × 10	5 × 10	5 × 10	5 × 10	5 × 10	5 × 10	5 × 8	5 × 8	5 × 8	5 × 8	5 × 8	5 × 8
Hang clean	127					4 × 4	4 × 3	4 × 3	3 × 3				
Romanian deadlift	67					4 × 6	4 × 6	4 × 6	2 × 6				
Bench press	55					3 × 6	3 × 6	3 × 5	3 × 4				
Glute–ham: bent knee	92					4 × 8	4 × 10	4 × 10	2 × 10				
Standing two-way calf raise	77					3 × 12	3 × 12	3 × 15	2 × 12				
Back squat	65									4 × 6	4 × 5	4 × 5	3 × 5
Push press	130									4 × 4	4 × 4	4 × 4	3 × 4
Seated row	57									3 × 8	3 × 6	3 × 6	2 × 6
Three-way weight transfer	77									3 × 10	3 × 10	3 × 10	2 × 10
General abs	169									Prog A	Prog A	Prog A	Prog A
Advanced abs	169					Prog B	Prog B	Prog B	Prog B				
High-intensity plyometrics	141									1-2 sest	2 sets	2 sets	1 set
Agility drills	118	1-2 sets	2 sets	2 sets	1 set								

Preseason 8-Week Program—Weeks 5 Through 8

Exercise	Page #	Monday				Wednesday				Friday			
		1	2	3	4	1	2	3	4	1	2	3	4
Power shrug	125	3 × 3	3 × 3	3 × 3	3 × 3								
Power clean	129	5 × 3	5 × 2	4 × 2	1RM					4 × 4	5 × 3	5 × 3	3 × 3
Back squat	65	5 × 3	5 × 3	4 × 2	1RM								
Bench press (incline)	55	3 × 5	3 × 4	3 × 4	3RM								
Forward box step-up	73	3 × 12	3 × 12	3 × 12									
Standing two-way calf raise	77	3 × 12	3 × 12	3 × 12		3 × 12	3 × 12	3 × 12					
Hang clean	127					4 × 3	4 × 3	4 × 2	1RM				
Front squat	66					5 × 4	5 × 3	4 × 2	1RM				
Bench press	55					3 × 3	3 × 3	3 × 2	1RM				
Glute–ham: bent knee	92					3 × 12	3 × 12	3 × 12					
Dumbbell rotator cuff routine	44					5 × 8	5 × 8	5 × 8	5 × 8	5 × 8	5 × 8	5 × 8	5 × 8
Back squat	65									4 × 5	4 × 5	4 × 5	3 × 5
Shoulder press (standing)	55									4 × 4	4 × 4	4 × 4	3 × 4
Lat pull-down	56									3 × 3	3 × 8	3 × 8	3 × 8
Three-way weight transfer bicep curl	76									3 × 10	3 × 10	3 × 10	3 × 10
General abs	169									Prog A	Prog A	Prog A	Prog A
Advanced abs	169					Prog B	Prog B	Prog B	Prog B				
High-intensity plyometrics	141									1-2 sets	2 sets	2 sets	1 set
Agility drills	118	1-2 sets	2 sets	2 sets	1 set								

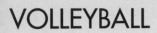

In-Season Maintenance 4-Week Program—Weeks 1 Through 4

Exercise	Page #	Monday 1	Monday 2	Monday 3	Monday 4	Wednesday 1	Wednesday 2	Wednesday 3	Wednesday 4
Power clean	129	3 × 3	3 × 3	3 × 2	3 × 3				
Back squat	65	3 × 4	3 × 4	3 × 3	2 × 4				
Bench press (incline)	55	3 × 6	3 × 5	3 × 4	3 × 3				
Dumbbell rotator cuff routine	44	5 × 8	5 × 8	5 × 8	5 × 8	5 × 6	5 × 6	5 × 6	5 × 6
Hang clean	127					3 × 3	3 × 3	3 × 2	3 × 2
Front squat	66					3 × 6	3 × 5	3 × 4	3 × 3
Bench press	55					3 × 4	3 × 4	3 × 3	3 × 3
Glute–ham: bent knee	92					3 × 12	3 × 12	3 × 12	3 × 8
Advanced abs	169					Prog B	Prog B	Prog B	Prog B
Moderate-intensity plyometrics	136	1-2 sets	2 sets	2 sets	1 set				

References and Resources

Books

Baechle, Thomas R., and Roger Earle. 2000. *Essentials of Strength Training and Conditioning, 2nd ed.* Champaign, IL: Human Kinetics.

Bompa, Tudor. 1997. *Power Training for Sport.* Oakville, Ontario: Mosaic.

Bompa, Tudor. 1999. *Periodization Training for Sports.* Champaign, IL: Human Kinetics.

Bompa, Tudor, Mauro Di Pasquale, and Lorenzo Cornacchia. 2003. *Serious Strength Training, 2nd ed.* Champaign, IL: Human Kinetics.

Chu, Donald A. 1998. *Jumping into Plyometrics.* Champaign, IL: Human Kinetics.

Delavier, Frédéric. 2003. *Women's Strength Training Anatomy.* Champaign, IL: Human Kinetics.

Fleck, Steven, and William Kraemer. 1996. *Periodization Breakthrough.* Ronkonkoma, NY: Advanced Research.

Johnson, Anne J., and Donna Lopiano. 1996. *Great Women in Sports.* Canton, MI: Visible Ink.

Kraemer, William J., and Keijo Hakkinen (Eds.). 2002. *Strength Training for Sport.* Oxford: Blackwell Scientific.

Kraemer, William J., and Steven Fleck. 1993. *Strength Training for Young Athletes.* Champaign, IL: Human Kinetics.

Newton, Harvey. 2002. *Explosive Lifting for Sports.* Champaign, IL: Human Kinetics.

Powe-Allred, Alexandra, and Michelle Powe. 1998. *The Quiet Storm: A Celebration of Women in Sport.* Chicago: Masters.

Warren, Michelle P., and Mona M. Shangold. 1997. *Sports Gynecology.* Oxford: Blackwell Scientific.

Zatsiorsky, Vladimir M. 1995. *Science and Practice of Strength Training.* Champaign, IL: Human Kinetics.

Audiotapes and Videotapes

Bengsbo, Jens. 1996. *Yo-Yo Tests for Soccer.* Audio tapes and booklet. Contact www.soccerfitness.com/yoyo.htm.

Boyle, Mike. 1998. *Stabilizing and Strengthening the Body's Torso.* Videotape. Cranston, RI: M-F Athletic Co; Perform Better Division.

Internet Resources

National Strength and Conditioning Association www.nsca-lift.org

American College of Sports Medicine www.acsm.org

National Athletic Trainers Association www.nata.org

American Physical Therapy Association www.apta.org

Index

Note: The italicized *f* and *t* following page numbers refer to figures and tables, respectively.

lower extremity. *See also specific muscles*
  anatomy of 61–64, 62t, 63f
  exercises for
    basic strength 64–71
    functional strength 72–77
    goals of 64
    warm-up 153–156, 160, 163
  injuries to 59–61
  testing 25–28
lumbar muscles. *See* back muscles
lunges
  power 73
  side 75
  stretches 153–154
  walking 72, 110

M
macrocycles 6, 6f
maximal heart rate (HRmax) 5
medicine ball exercises
  in abdominals and core training programs 169t
  chest pass 93, 104
  extended crunch 104
  overhead throw 95, 104
  twist pass 94
menisci 61–62
mesocycles 6, 6t
microcycles 6, 7f
mile run 33
mode of training, defined 5
multidirectional speed. *See* agility
multijoint exercises, defined 65
muscles
  core 79–82, 81t, 82f
  lower extremity 62–64, 62t, 63f
  shoulder 40f, 41–42, 41t
muscle soreness, reducing 150
muscular endurance
  defined 16
  exercises for 117
  testing 33–35

N
neural patterns, correcting 81
no-step vertical leap 25

O
off-season training. *See also specific sports*
  core training in 83–84, 83t
  described 7–8
  plyometrics in 144t–145t
  testing and 15
Olympic weightlifting
  lifts 124–130
  as mode of training 5
one-step vertical leap 26
overhead side raise 48
overhead throw, medicine ball 95, 104
overspeed training 115–116
overtraining, avoiding 4, 9
overuse injuries
  avoiding 150
  hips 81
  shoulder 43

P
partner chest stretch 157
pectoralis

exercises for
  strengthening 54, 55
  warm-up 157, 161
  in shoulder anatomy 40f, 41t
periodization
  age-appropriate 11–14
  approaches to 4
  of core training 83, 83t
  defined 4
  phases in 5–10, 6f, 6t
  of plyometrics program 132t
  variables in 4–5
physioball swimmer 58
pike 98
pillars 96
piriformis
  in core anatomy 80, 81t
  in lower-extremity anatomy 62t, 63, 63f
play, as exercise 11–12
plyometrics
  described 123, 131
  exercises
    high-intensity 141–142
    low-intensity 133–135
    moderate-intensity 136–140
    off-season program for 144t–145t
  periodization scheme for 132t
  safety considerations for 131–132
  for upper-body 143
postadolescent training 13–14
posterior muscles, in shoulder 40f, 41, 41t
postseason training 10
power
  defined 16–17
  exercises for 93–95, 117
  testing 25–28
power clean 129
power lunge 73
power push-up 56
power shrug 125
power skip 111
prayer and seal stretches 158
prepubescent training 12–13
preschool-age training 11–12
preseason training. *See also specific sports*
  core training in 83–84, 83t
  described 9
  speed and agility training in 120–122, 121t, 170t
proprioception
  defined 8
  exercises for 93–96, 104
  testing 27
pull-up test 33
push press 130
push-ups
  bridge 97
  forearm 52
  handstand 56
  power 56
  test 34

Q
Q-angles 60
quadratus femoris
  in core anatomy 80, 81t
  in lower-extremity anatomy 62t, 63, 63f

quadratus lumborum 79–80, 81t, 82f
quadriceps
  exercises for
    strengthening 66, 69–70, 72–74, 76–77, 110
    warm-up 155, 162–163
  in knee injuries 60
  in lower-extremity anatomy 62t, 63, 63f
quadriceps angles (Q-angles) 60
quadriceps stretch 155
quality of training 10
quick-response jump 135

R
range-of-motion exercises 158–161
RDL 67
recovery and adaptation 4
repetition maximum (RM) 5
repetitions, defined 4
resistance machines, versus free weights 12, 13
rest and recovery
  defined 5
  in in-season training 10
  in training program 14
reverse crunch 90
reverse hyperextension 101
rhomboids
  exercises for 57
  in shoulder anatomy 40f
rhythm 108
rice: three way 58
RM 5
Romanian deadlift (RDL) 67
rotator cuff muscles
  anatomy of 40f, 41, 41t
  exercises for
    strengthening 44–51
    warm-up 160–161
running evaluation form 110t
running form 109
running speed 107

S
sartorius
  in core anatomy 80, 81t
  in lower-extremity anatomy 62t, 63, 63f
scapula 39–41, 40f
scapular stabilizers, exercises for 52–54, 57
SC joint 40, 40f, 41
seated row 67
serratus, exercises for 52–54
sets, defined 4
shin angles 109
shoulder flexion, 45-degree 45
shoulder press 55
shoulders
  anatomy of 39–42, 40f, 41t
  exercises for
    body-weight shoulder stabilization routine 52–54
    dumbbell rotator cuff routine 44–51
    upper-extremity strengtheners 55–58
  functions of 42
  injuries to 8, 43
shuffle squat 77

About the Authors

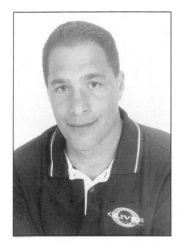

David Oliver is the president and founder of Oliver Sports Performance. He has worked at the high school, collegiate, professional, and Olympic levels as a coach and athletic trainer for more than 15 years. He has worked as the conditioning coach for the U.S. women's national soccer team and served as strength and conditioning consultant to the U.S. women's national basketball team. He has served as an athletic trainer on medical teams assembled for major events like the U.S. National Skating Championships, the World Triathlon Championships, the Citrus Bowl, and the NBA All-Star Game.

Oliver also spent seven years with the NBA's Orlando Magic basketball team as the strength and conditioning coach and assistant athletic trainer. Oliver is a certified member of the National Athletic Trainers' Association (NATA), the National Strength and Conditioning Association (NSCA), and the American College of Sports Medicine (ACSM). He is also certified as a U.S. Weightlifting Federation (USWF) club coach. He speaks nationally at camps, clinics, and seminars and is well regarded for his innovative training techniques.

Oliver is the coauthor of *Conditioning the NBA Way* and *NBA Power Conditioning* and has written articles for *Men's Health*, *Men's Journal*, *Women's Health and Fitness*, and numerous other publications. He has also been featured in *Women's Sports Illustrated* and *Conditioning for Women's Basketball*.

He lives with his wife, Shelly, and sons Zachary and Ryan in Orlando, Florida.

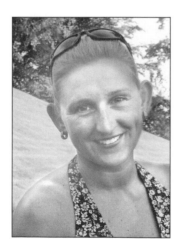

Dana Healy is the department head for strength and conditioning at the United States Olympic Committee (USOC). In this position she oversees the strength and conditioning programs at three Olympic Training Centers (OTCs) and consults with teams that do not reside at the OTCs. She has been with the USOC since 1997 and has trained numerous Olympic and world medalists.

Before joining the USOC, Healy worked as the assistant strength coach at Brown University. She is a certified member of the National Strength and Conditioning Association (NSCA), the American College of Sports Medicine (ACSM), and USA Weightlifting (USAW) and has been a contributor to *Men's Health*, *Outside Magazine*, *Sports Illustrated for Women*, and *Performance Conditioning*.

Healy lives in Colorado Springs, Colorado.

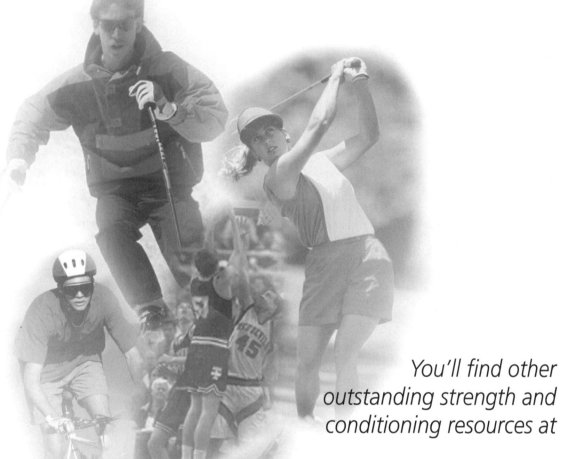